The
Alzheimer's
Epidemic

Searching for Causes and a Cure

Danton H. O'Day, PhD

Published by eBookIt.com

ISBN-13: 978-1-4566-1641-0

About the Cover

The picture on the cover is an original work by Ronald P. Falcioni titled "Synapse". This dynamic work suggests the explosive and complex events that occur at brain synapses that ultimately become diminished with the onset and progression of Alzheimer's disease.

Dedication

To Susan, my patient and loving wife, who as an RN has served on the front-lines of eldercare and Alzheimer's disease counseling. Her advice, insightful guidance and encouragement were central to the completion of this book.

Acknowledgements

I would like to thank Dr. Robert Huber, Harvard Medical School, for his critical and helpful comments. I owe a great deal of thanks to Aldona Budniak who gave many constructive comments and provided invaluable editing as the book was being written. Last, I would like to thank my life-long friend Ronald Falcioni who not only provided the cover picture but who also gave some valuable encouragement. Any errors or omissions are my sole responsibility and I welcome readers to inform me of any that they may find.

Danton H. O'Day, PhD
Oakville, ON, CANADA

TABLE OF CONTENTS

Tau Phosphorylation: Identifying the Culprits
Tangling Tau: A Complex Web of Kinases
Tau and the Mind of a Mouse
Tau Can Move from Neuron to Neuron

The Major Hypotheses for Alzheimer's Disease
The Yin-Yang of Plaque Formation as a Target
Amyloid Hypothesis-Based Drugs
Beta-Secretase as a Pharmaceutical Target
The Continuing Search for Secretase Inhibitors
Will New Beta-Secretase Inhibitors Ride to the Rescue?
Treatments Targeting Tau
Many Kinases Turn Good Tau Bad
Drugs that Prevent or Reduce Tangles
Why Do Some Promising Drugs Fail?

The Cholinergic Hypothesis
Therapies Based on Acetylcholine
Acetylcholinesterase Inhibitors
FDA-Approved Cholinergic Drugs
Clinical Variations Can Hide Information

Glutamate and NMDA Receptors
NMDA Receptors as Pharmacological Targets
Memantine as an Alzheimer's Drug
NMDA Receptors and Neuron Death

Biomarkers and Their Uses
The Search for Causes and Predictors
Required Attributes of Biomarkers
Biochemical Biomarkers: Assessing Preclinical Stages
Tracking the Movements of Amyloid Beta
Other Biochemical Markers of Alzheimer's

Brain Imaging as a Biomarker
Magnetic Resonance Imaging (MRI)
Episodic versus Semantic Memory
Functional versus Structural MRI
PET Scans
Sugar for Your PET
EEG: Electrical Imaging of the Alzheimer's Brain
Cognitive Self-Testing for Alzheimer's Disease
Formal Cognitive Screening
The Biomarker Future
Alzheimer's May Start Decades before Any Symptoms

Genetic Links to Alzheimer's Disease
Down Syndrome and Alzheimer's Disease
The Link to Tangle Formation
Three Bad Genes Linked to Early-Onset Alzheimer's
Some Good News: Gene Mutation Defends Against Alzheimer's
Late-Onset Susceptibility Genes
Good Genes Can Do Bad Things
APOE: A Cholesterol-Associated Protein Linked to Alzheimer's

Putting Amyloid Beta in the Garbage Instead of in Plaques
Nine Offenders with Unfriendly Names
PICALM Stands Out in One Study
GWAS: Genome-Wide Association Studies

Dealing with Symptoms versus Causes
Why is it Taking So Long?
Stages of Drug Development
Scientist versus Clinician versus Patient: Different Points of View
The Problems Facing Alzheimer's Drug Research
Analyzing Drug Success Is an Issue
A New Drug for Detecting Plaques

Preface

The "Alzheimer's Epidemic" has begun. As the number of aged individuals worldwide continues to grow the epidemic will continue unabated. Alzheimer's disease will affect one in three families. In addition to the devastating implications of this epidemic to Alzheimer's sufferers, their families and caregivers, the economic costs to society will be enormous. Around the world governments are struggling with ways to deal with this unrelenting tide that will soon be a medical tsunami that will challenge many societies' ability to cope. At the front of this attempt to stem the tide are biomedical researchers worldwide who are working diligently to understand the causes of Alzheimer's, which will allow them to formulate ways to slow the progression of the disease and someday stop it from occurring.

This book looks at this "Alzheimer's Epidemic" by focusing on the causes and the search for a cure. Other books have dealt in detail with the symptoms of the disease and how to care for those suffering with the disease. I have done research on the proteins linked to the onset and progression of Alzheimer's disease and have written several articles on the subject. This book is significantly different from those that have gone before. The content is gleaned from original research and reviews including recent international meetings. With my strong science background, I have tried to write the book in a way that will appeal to the non-scientist reader so citations within the text are avoided. Instead, the reader is directed to the selected list of references at the end of the book. There is also a list of websites that can provide information on the very latest advances in Alzheimer's research.

At times it is essential to delve into the nitty-gritty of the relevant science. So this book takes the reader well beyond what they can glean from newspapers and magazines. It sets the stage for an in-depth understanding of what is being done and where research is going in the quest to understand the causes and find a cure for Alzheimer's disease.

Danton H. O'Day
Oakville, Ontario, CANADA

Chapter 1

Introduction and Overview

As we progress through the 21st century, the world will be faced with a population dominated by an increasing number of elderly people. Since older individuals often do not work outside the home and have significantly more health issues, the impact on society will be immense. This isn't their fault, because aging is a fact of life. What is, or more correctly will be, at fault is society's failure to address the issues raised by this aging population. The goal of this book is to look at a single aspect of aging: The Alzheimer's Epidemic. In this introductory chapter, we will detail and put into perspective material that will be covered in the book.

The scenarios that the media puts out about our senescing population are sometimes frightening. Old folks, it seems, are going to be a major negative drain on society in a number of ways, not the least of which is living longer and draining funds from old-age pensions. Thus, Alzheimer's disease (AD) isn't the only medical problem that faces the aged. The cumulative effect of all of these problems will become a serious issue for society in the future, leading to major medical costs for healthcare and increasing the need for long-term residential accommodation. It might seem a bit incongruous, then, to be looking for ways to improve the health and extend the life of seniors—but curing, stopping or slowing a single disease such as Alzheimer's will have major benefits on a multitude of levels to Alzheimer's sufferers, their families, caregivers and society.

The Alzheimer's Epidemic

Before we begin, we need to get things clear up front. Just what is The Alzheimer's Epidemic? How can a disease like Alzheimer's be considered an epidemic? Typically we think of an epidemic as a disease caused by a viral or bacterial infection. However, an epidemic can also be considered to be the widespread occurrence of a disease that greatly surpasses what would normally be expected.

Alzheimer's disease can be considered an epidemic because it is widespread and continues to spread very rapidly. While it is not caused by a contagious agent, there is one known direct cause of Alzheimer's disease: that cause is aging. There is an unprecedented growth of elderly populations worldwide. According to the US Centers for Disease Control and Prevention, the World Health Organization and the United Nations, this is due not only to the aging of the current population but also to the decline in fertility that is occurring around the world. Thus people are getting older while fewer children are being born.

Things are going to get a lot worse before they get better and the cost to society could be potentially unsustainable. At best, the cost will drain medical resources of all but those countries with the most robust economies. So there is an unquestionable need not only to find a cure but, in the short term, to find ways to diminish the effects of the disease. This is most evident on the frontlines of the disease: the impact on the individual and their immediate family.

The word "dementia" used to be an alternative term for madness. Today dementia is defined as a significant decline in one's mental functioning. This intellectual decline can involve problems with thinking, reasoning and memory. Alzheimer's is the most common form of dementia in that it accounts for between 50–70% of all dementia cases. It is estimated that Alzheimer's disease affects one in eight people who are over 65 years old. The incidence increases with age so that about 42% of individuals over 85 years old are afflicted with the disease. Already the impact of Alzheimer's worldwide is staggering—more than 24 million people are suffering from the disease.

The problem is these numbers are increasing with a new case of Alzheimer's disease occurring every 7 seconds. Based on statistical analyses of our aging populations, it is projected that the number of Alzheimer's sufferers will double every 20 years. Thus there is no doubt that the disease is on the verge of truly reaching epidemic proportions with devastating implications to societies worldwide. The Alzheimer's crisis has started and scientists are trying to deal with it. It has been argued that if the onset of Alzheimer's disease can be delayed by a single year through therapeutic intervention then there would be around nine million fewer cases than expected by 2050!

Thus, with a new case being diagnosed every seven seconds worldwide, Alzheimer's disease is on the brink of reaching devastating epidemic proportions as the world population ages and more sufferers appear. Is this a stoppable epidemic or one that will drain our personal and societal resources both emotionally and financially? At present, with no cure on the horizon, the epidemic seems all the more daunting.

To add to this concern, at present there are no drugs that can stop the progression of the disease. Those that are available can alleviate the symptoms of Alzheimer's but only for a limited time. Why is this? It is because no one truly understands what causes the disease. While many of the symptoms and the phases of progression of the disease are known, what precipitates Alzheimer's disease remains a mystery. As we will see, even the suspects that are believed to cause the neurological degeneration that occurs in Alzheimer's disease in fact may not be the initial cause of the disease. Will we end up spending billions of dollars investigating the wrong culprits?

This book is not designed to offer false hope. It is designed to offer realistic hope—and there is hope. This volume aims to give hope by explaining what we do know about the onset, development and progression of Alzheimer's disease. It will reveal the primary targets of research and exactly what is being done to knock out those targets. It will provide hope by showing that all of the past research has not been in vain—it has set the stage for a successful future. Inroads are being made into this complex and, as yet, poorly understood disease. Hope lies on the horizon—just how far away that horizon is remains to be determined. This chapter will provide an overview of subjects and issues that subsequent chapters will deal with in detail. So let's begin with a look at what the disease is and what are believed to be the primary causes.

Three Types of Alzheimer's Disease

The two major delineations of Alzheimer's disease are based on when the symptoms of the disease appear while the third is due to a chromosomal defect (Figure 1.1). The predominant form of Alzheimer's disease occurs in people after the age of 65. It is called late-onset Alzheimer's disease or LOAD, an acronym used by workers in the field. A smaller proportion of sufferers fall into the category of early-onset Alzheimer's disease, which some refer to as EOAD. In other words, early-onset sufferers are people who get Alzheimer's prior to age 65 and typically at a much younger age. The early-onset cohort has allowed researchers to find certain genes that are linked to the disease, as detailed in Chapter 12. The early-onset form of the disease contributes to about 10–15% of Alzheimer's cases and usually begins in one's 50s or 60s but can occur earlier in life. The third group of Alzheimer's disease individuals comes from those with Down syndrome. Down syndrome individuals develop Alzheimer's at a comparatively early age: symptoms often appear around the mid-40s, with the average age of diagnosis being in the mid-50s. Just as important, the disease progresses rapidly in those with the syndrome.

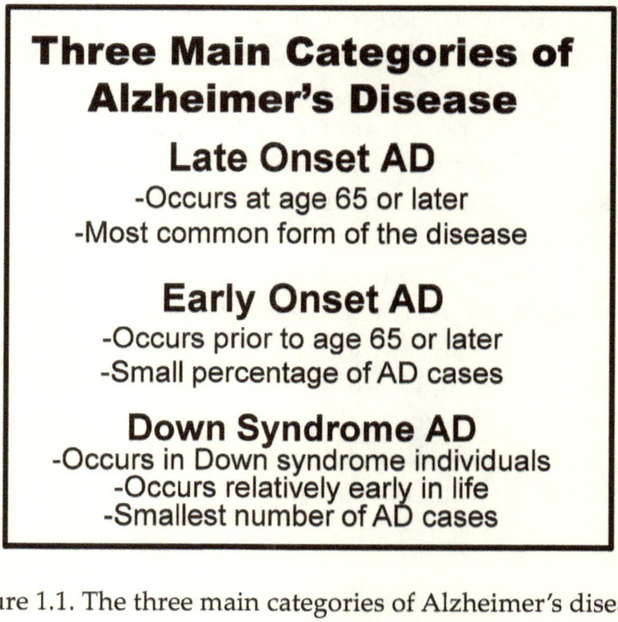

Three Main Categories of Alzheimer's Disease

Late Onset AD
-Occurs at age 65 or later
-Most common form of the disease

Early Onset AD
-Occurs prior to age 65 or later
-Small percentage of AD cases

Down Syndrome AD
-Occurs in Down syndrome individuals
-Occurs relatively early in life
-Smallest number of AD cases

Figure 1.1. The three main categories of Alzheimer's disease.

While there is a clear genetic basis for the onset of Alzheimer's disease in Down syndrome persons, as clarified in Chapter 12, this can't be used to explain the late- or early-onset forms of the disease that occur in non-Down-syndrome individuals. The bottom line is, while each form of the disease can provide insight, they are fundamentally different. To add to this complexity, the signs and symptoms of Alzheimer's disease vary markedly from person to person. This has prompted some researchers to argue Alzheimer's is not a disease but a syndrome. In this volume we will cover all forms of the disease with a primary focus on late-onset Alzheimer's disease because it is the cause of the largest number of cases of the disease—it is the primary cause of the Alzheimer's epidemic.

Fighting the Odds

There is no guarantee that you can avoid Alzheimer's disease. While early-onset Alzheimer's disease begins to appear before the age of 65, late-onset Alzheimer's disease typically occurs long after 65 years of age. As detailed in Chapter 12 in this book, the early-onset form is primarily driven by inheritance. It is due to mutations in three different genes that lead to abnormal levels of amyloid beta peptide. In contrast, late-onset Alzheimer's disease has not been proven to be caused by specific gene mutations; while there are genetic links, it appears to be a result of the combination of aging and lifestyle among other contributing factors. Thus, eating a healthy, well-balanced diet is one thing a person can do to decrease the odds of developing the late-onset form of the disease. Coupling this with regular exercise and avoiding a sedentary lifestyle can also help. Using one's brain actively in various activities like crossword puzzles, Sudoku, etc. is believed to help stave off memory decline. As you might expect, passively watching shows on TV is less than beneficial.

Lifestyles and Alzheimer's Disease

While medical researchers define stages of Alzheimer's, the development of the disease doesn't involve a stepwise sequence of events. It is a continuum that begins with mild cognitive issues and can progress resulting in severe cognitive defects and dementia. So when an individual begins to show signs that might suggest changes in their ability to remember or reason, this doesn't mean that this will immediately lead to the next step which would be much more severe. In fact, mild cognitive issues may not progress at all. If they do, their rate of progression can vary markedly from individual to individual. Thus it is important to understand the significance of lifestyle in the onset and progression of Alzheimer's disease as well as other cognitive diseases. But remember, while you can do all the right things to decrease the odds that you will suffer from Alzheimer's disease, there is no guarantee that doing so will help you avoid the disease. That is why we need to develop improved methods for detecting, slowing and one day stopping the disease.

We All Forget Things but Alzheimer's Is Different

We all forget things. Where did we put our keys? What's the name of this person I just bumped into in the mall? These are short-term memory losses everyone faces—but what would it be like to forget everything? To forget the people we love? To not remember where we live? To not know who we are? As if that's not bad enough, there is also the loss of the ability to reason. Ultimately all communication with the world around you can be lost. These are some of the effects of Alzheimer's disease—a progressive and irretrievable loss of memory, a slow descent into a new world that cannot be understood.

We all know when we have forgotten something or can't remember something else. But what do we do when we can't remember what we've forgotten? Where do our memories go when we develop Alzheimer's disease? Do they go to a place so hidden away that they can't be found? Or do they remain in the same place but the route to finding them is gone, like a lost treasure map? Is it more basic than that? Do our memories simply get erased? Are they completely removed so they can never be remembered again?

All of these possibilities are the product of brain activity that is progressively lost as Alzheimer's disease onsets and progresses to full-fledged dementia. Since the brain is an organ, it is made up of cells. A large number of these cells are specialized nerve cells or neurons. Neurons, through their interactions with other neurons and other cells in the brain, serve to process incoming information and to store this information as the basis of our memories. Thus, in one way or another, our memories are stored within cells in our brains. Because neurons are the primary unit of brain function, Alzheimer's disease can be considered a disease of brain cells.

Cells of the Alzheimer's Brain

As we will see in Chapter 5, the brain is actually made up of many types of cells but it is the neurons that are of primary interest in Alzheimer's disease because it is these cells that show the first clear evidence of the disease. The brain neurons are the central place where the changes of the Alzheimer's brain begin and end. As a result, they are the site where scientists hope to find the cure for Alzheimer's disease. Searching the brain for the cause of Alzheimer's is much like an episode of the television show CSI; it is a true Crime Scene Investigation. Rather than investigating a dying person, we are essentially looking at the slow death of the brain—the site of all reason, learning and memory. So, like a crime scene, we want to see what is different from the normal brain as compared to the Alzheimer's brain. Then we want to understand how those differences arose: what caused a good brain to go bad. Finally, when we understand what caused the disease, we want to learn how to prevent it. But science and crime scene investigation are like life: sometimes the culprit is elusive and evades detection or capture. In that case, we have to compromise. Since we can't prevent the death of the brain, we want to at least be able to slow its degeneration or, even better, stop it in its tracks. This approach will have to do until the cause or biochemical culprits responsible for Alzheimer's disease are finally found and scientists can begin to prevent the disease, slow it or, hopefully, develop a cure.

So that's what we're going to do in the book. We're going to see what we know about the underlying events of Alzheimer's disease as it relates to brain cells. What causes these brain cells to lose their ability to function properly? What causes them to die? How can we slow this sequence of events? And, ultimately, how can we determine how the disease starts? Before we get out our microscopes and our biochemical tools to understand these changes, let's look at a short history of Alzheimer's disease to understand how this disease was first identified and how that discovery set the stage for how things sit today.

A Very Short History of Alzheimer's Disease

Unofficially, Alzheimer's disease has been around as long as human beings have existed as thinking entities. It didn't become an official disease until it was properly diagnosed by Alois Alzheimer. Dr. Alzheimer described the behavioral characteristics of Alzheimer's disease over 100 years ago, which in itself was a major medical advancement. His work, however, went much further. He also delved into the underlying changes in the brain that were associated with the disease. To this day, his prescience defined the three primary neurological attributes of Alzheimer's disease: the appearance of senile plaque and tangles coupled with the death of brain cells (Figure 1.2). These are still the primary criteria that are used today for defining the disease. As such, while plaques and tangles are introduced later in this chapter and will be covered throughout this volume, they are presented in much greater detail in Chapters 6 and 7.

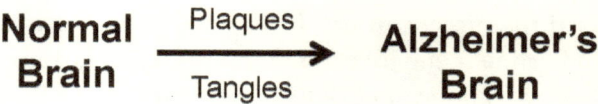

Figure 1.2. Alois Alzheimer discovered the primary hallmarks of Alzheimer's disease: plaques and tangles.

The Personal Side of Alzheimer's Disease

What is Alzheimer's disease? This might sound like a simple question to answer but it is not. This is because this disease is different things to different people. To a clinician or biomedical researcher, it is the buildup of bad stuff in the brain, the loss of specific nerve cells or changes in cognitive behavior. To a doctor, it's the emotional challenge of having to diagnose a person with the disease and telling them they can no longer do the things they want to do. To a caregiver, it's a 24-hour-a-day challenge without a positive outcome. To a family member, it's the loss of the person they knew and loved. To the Alzheimer's sufferer, it begins with the loss of their memory and dignity and ends with the loss of their whole world. To anyone who has seen the face of Alzheimer's, all of these points of view are important because they all play a part in helping us understand this devastating disease. So let's start with the currently held view of how the disease starts and progresses. Then, as we work our way through this book, we will develop this knowledge into the full picture of Alzheimer's disease as it is understood today.

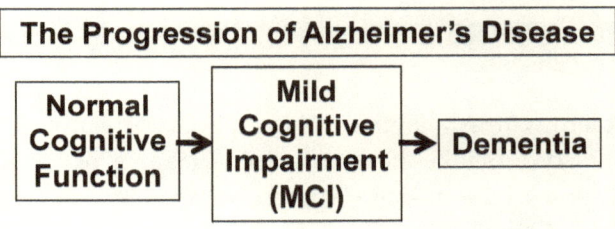

Figure 1.3. The basic stages in the progression of Alzheimer's disease.

Alzheimer's disease involves a progressive loss of mental ability that begins with mild cognitive impairment (i.e., decreased ability to think, reason, remember), or MCI, that can progress, in the worst case, to true dementia (Figure 1.3). One of the problems in research has been that different biomedical researchers and clinicians have formulated a diversity of stages and sub-stages for the disease. While these are well intentioned and of value for the researcher, they make it more difficult to discuss the disease in lay terms. So in this book, except when absolutely needed, the disease will be discussed in terms of mild cognitive impairment occurring as a prelude to dementia.

As we age our ability to remember things declines gradually. In Alzheimer's disease, this decline is often more rapid and more devastating. Rather than symptoms like forgetting a name or the inability to immediately remember it, the disease is reflected in more severe memory impairment. Initially the memory loss is mild but worse than a normal individual of the same age and health. As it progresses, the person who is afflicted may not even realize where they are, even when in their own home or neighborhood. They may not recognize family members and friends. By the time the disease has affected a person's ability to function socially or to continue in their job, they are in the clinical stage of dementia.

Alzheimer's disease is a cruel affliction that progressively robs a person's sense of self and awareness. Following a pathway to cognitive oblivion, it turns loved ones and friends into strangers and, at its worst, enemies. The very world in which the Alzheimer's sufferer lives becomes foreign if not frightening, as altered brain cells slowly erase that person's past and their grip on reality. Then those brain cells die, signaling the final stages of this horrific disease.

The problem with Alzheimer's disease is that it is not like typical medical disorders like heart disease, diabetes or even cancer. Those diseases have specific symptoms that, for the most part, are clearly definable. In most cases, medical intervention and well-defined approaches for a cure are available. The course of these diseases is also fairly predictable. This is not the case with Alzheimer's. There are multiple pathologies associated with the disease. The disease is person specific and doesn't follow a predictable pathway. There are no available cures and even attempts to slow the disease are not well developed.

The Reality of Alzheimer's Disease

No matter how you slice it, Alzheimer's is a devastating disease that wreaks havoc on the lives of individuals and their families. We notice that, as we age, it can be difficult to remember a work or a name. As a senior, I was shocked when I was playing Mario Kart on my Nintendo with my grandson. I thought I was doing quite well motoring along, dropping a few banana peels and turtle shells to slow his progress. But I was 100% focused on controlling my car. The game was all I could concentrate on. Meanwhile, my grandson was not only doing everything I was doing, he was giving me hints on things I could do as well as carrying on a conversation with three other people in the room. If that didn't demonstrate to me the loss of cognitive ability I was suffering, nothing could.

But Alzheimer's disease presents itself as more than a short-term loss of memory or forgetfulness, it begins with a major loss in one's ability to recall and reason. More importantly, it can progress to the state were the sufferer is often confused about where they are or what they are doing. It can cause them to forget who their loved ones are. Having said this, the disease is not something that is a natural extension of growing old. Also, the progression from loss of memory to full-fledged dementia is not a given. Understanding exactly what separates simple loss of memory from aging versus true Alzheimer's disease is important and will become much clearer as the reader progresses through this volume.

You, Your Family and Alzheimer's Disease

It's tough to worry about the world around you and what the future will bring when you or someone close to you has developed Alzheimer's disease. While the implications of losing one's touch with reality are overwhelming, the disease has other wide-ranging effects. It decreases the quality of life not only for the sufferer but also for family members, for whom the impact is equally devastating. One's own family is the predominant cornerstone for the care of the Alzheimer's sufferer. For example, it has been estimated that in Canada the psychological impact of having the responsibility of being the primary caregiver is immense. Between 40 and 70% of caregivers have been shown to experience psychological problems because of the pressures they face in having to assist someone with the disease. With 15–30% of caregivers, these responsibilities led to full clinical depression. There is little doubt that these numbers can be extrapolated to family caregivers worldwide. The number of hours family caregivers lovingly sacrifice is great and increases as the disease continues to progress in the family member they care for. In Canada, the total time dedicated to caring for family members with the disease will approach 800 million hours per year. When this is coupled with annual healthcare costs reaching up to 150 billion dollars within the next 25–30 years, it becomes clear why we are facing a true Alzheimer's epidemic.

Healthcare Workers and Alzheimer's Disease

The frontline workers who deal with Alzheimer's disease are nurses and other healthcare workers who strive daily to make the patients' and their families' lives more bearable and livable. With the loss of the persons' intellectual awareness, harmful prejudices, real and imagined, rise to the surface. In the worst cases, physical violence can accompany verbal assault. In spite of this, healthcare workers must rise above such routine onslaughts to their person, race or beliefs. This aspect of the disease and the toll it takes on caregivers of all stripes is rarely recognized by family members whose primary focus is on their sibling, father, mother or grandparent. It is also of little concern to the person with the disease who often will be trying desperately to hang on to whatever reality remains in their lives. Through no fault of their own, they have lost the ability to separate appropriate from inappropriate behavior. We forget too that the healthcare worker is bound by laws and legalities that are designed to meet the needs of the many while often ignoring their own safety and mental health. Typically the last ones considered are those who deliver patient care. These are just some of the unquantifiable costs of the disease. So like a stone thrown into a pond, the behavioral effects of Alzheimer's disease start from the patient, rippling ever outward, disrupting the calm waters of whomever resides in that human pond.

Quality of Life: An Important Issue

As the disease progresses, the quality of life of the Alzheimer's sufferer will diminish. However there are aspects that friends and family can take into account to improve the individual's quality of life. There are things that should be done and things that should not be done. Some of these are summarized in the following graph which gives some indication of factors that can improve the quality of life for those afflicted with Alzheimer's disease (Figure 1.4).

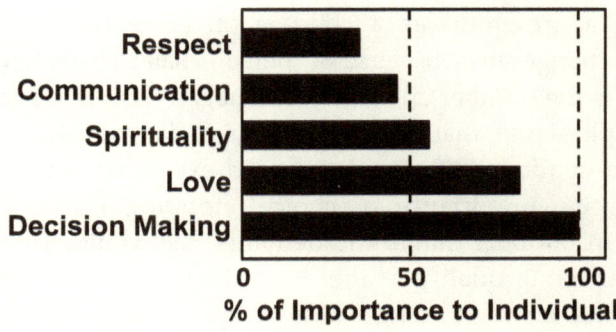

Figure 1.4. Things that can improve the quality of life. Data from Banerjee, S. et al, 2010a,b.

Thus it is clear that being allowed to make their own decisions is paramount to the individual with Alzheimer's disease. Being able to make their own choices can improve their quality of life. Being loved by the ones they care for, or cared about, is also a major element in ensuring a good quality of life. Spirituality, clear communication and respect are also important overall but less so than love and decision making. If we look at the other side of the coin, then we can see issues that diminish the quality of life for the person with Alzheimer's. Just as the former elements make life better, the following make life worse: treating the individual as a child, emphasizing the disease itself, stopping them from doing things or making them do things. These are summarized in the following graph (Figure 1.5).

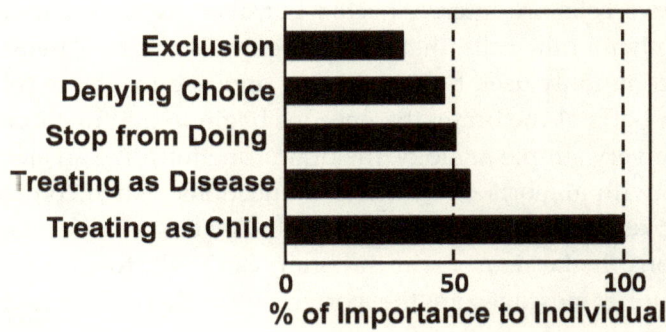

Figure 1.5. Things that can decrease the quality of life for the Alzheimer's disease sufferer. Data from Banerjee, S. et al, 2010a,b.

Treating a grown-up as a child is offensive to anyone. This doesn't change just because a person has Alzheimer's. This element is the number one factor that negatively affects quality of life. Emphasizing that the person has a disease also impinges badly on quality of life. As one would expect from the primary and positive importance of choice, stopping the Alzheimer's sufferer from doing things and denying them choice are negative factors affecting quality of life. Excluding them from joining in with others in day-to-day events or special occasions is also a negative factor. While exclusion apparently is less impactful than treating the person as child, it is still an important element.

Clearly the percentages given in the previous two graphs are somewhat arbitrary because they are based on the personal opinions of a diverse group. But they do serve as a guide. The key thing to remember is that quality of life comes from a package of these elements, not just one or two, or even three. For example, giving the person choice is of little value if that choice isn't given out of love and respect. The aforementioned issues are also not the only things that affect quality of life. So it is important to think about what different aspects of the individual's life are impacting the quality of that life and focus on improving those that are supportive while diminishing the negative elements.

Plaques and Tangles

How does this destruction of the Alzheimer's brain happen? All of our memories are stored in our brains, primarily in the way the nerve cells are interconnected but also via their interactions with other brain cells that are present. (The term "neuron" is more commonly used by scientists as opposed to "nerve cell".) In certain parts of the brain, the neurons begin to malfunction. If we make a very simple analogy, the brain functions like an electronic device with all sorts of electrical connections. When connections are broken, the device may fail or only be able to perform certain functions. If the neurons in the brain can't talk to each other or pass along messages in the correct way, then the brain can't operate correctly. With the progression of the disease, neurons also begin to die. When brain cells no longer communicate with each other, this can lead to their death. This cell death of neurons leads to brain shrinkage and actual "holes" in areas of the brain.

Your next question might be, "How do brain cells fail and die?" Since neurons and other brain cells fail and die in normal brains as well, this is an important question. In fact this cell death is a critical part of normal brain development *in utero*. In the embryo, millions more brain cells are made than are required. The excess cells are then killed off in an organized way by a process called "programmed cell death" (or, to use the appropriate scientific term, "apoptosis") that will be discussed later in the book. Brain cells are also killed throughout life. The death of brain cells is important in the building of the connections between them that define how our brain operates. This cell death also removes cells that are not essential for these normal brain functions.

With Alzheimer's disease, brain cell death is a concern because, unlike normal cell death in brains, it is uncontrolled and it occurs at an alarming rate over an extended period of time. Good brain cells are killed off indiscriminately. For now, we'll talk in generalities about the two major reasons why this occurs. Both of these reasons involve proteins (Figure 1.6). One of the reasons is the buildup of plaques outside of and between brain cells, a hallmark of Alzheimer's disease discovered by Alois Alzheimer. These plaques are made up of proteins of which one is the primary culprit. This very small protein culprit is called "amyloid beta". Actually, since it's a relatively short sequence of amino acids, it more correctly is called a peptide as detailed in Chapter 6. The amyloid beta peptide is secreted in large amounts by Alzheimer's neurons but not normal brain cells. Outside the cells, amyloid beta accumulates in plaques, large protein masses that surround brain cells and interfere with their function and survival. As a result, there is a direct correlation between the appearance of the protein in these plaques and the process of neurodegeneration.

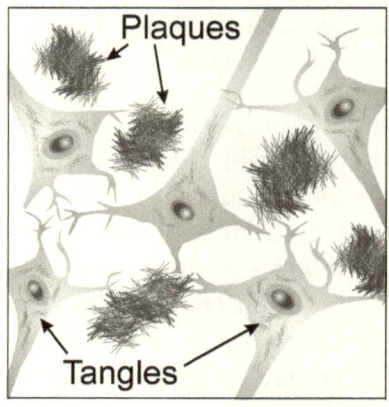

Figure 1.6. Protein deposits in the Alzheimer's brain. Plaques of amyloid beta peptide accumulate outside of brain cells, while neurofibrillary tangles made of tau protein localize inside them.

The second culprit that Alois Alzheimer identified is the fine tangles inside of the neurons of Alzheimer's brains. Like disorganized tangles of thread, these protein masses work inside of brain cells to negatively alter their function. The protein involved is tau, like the Greek letter. Tau works in normal cells but when large amounts accumulate and it is modified, as we'll discuss later in Chapter 7, it forms filamentous masses called neurofibrillary tangles.

So you might ask, "If amyloid beta and tau are so bad, why can't we just prevent their buildup in the brain?" That's where the story gets a bit more complicated. So we'll come back to this later in the book. But be aware that tens of thousands of researchers worldwide are trying to figure out just how amyloid beta and tau work and how to stop them from doing what they do.

The Search for Biomarkers

Biomarkers are indicators of the existence of or the potential for developing a specific disease. The quest for biomarkers is of central interest to biomedical researchers in all fields. A biomarker may be the presence of a certain component in the blood or some other bodily fluid. For atherosclerosis, bad cholesterol is a biomarker—an indicator that the individual with high blood LDL (low-density lipoprotein) is on the pathway to ill health. For prostate cancer, PSA (prostate-specific antigen) is often used as a biomarker. A biomarker can also be a behavioral, psychological or physiological indicator as we will cover later in this volume. By knowing what biomarker is best for determining if a specific disease is present, doctors can then assess the situation, determine the risk and help their patients accordingly.

So what is the biomarker? Actually there is more than one current biomarker for Alzheimer's disease and others are being searched for even as you read this chapter. In Chapter 11 we'll talk about this quest for biomarkers. For now, let's look at the prime candidates. To do this we need to look mainly at two events we've already touched upon: the appearance of amyloid plaques and neurofibrillary tangles. Let's start with the plaques.

As discussed above, we know that amyloid plaques form outside of nerve cells in the brain and are tightly linked to the development and progress of Alzheimer's disease. Most researchers believe this accumulation of amyloid peptides and other proteins in those plaques is a primary cause of Alzheimer's disease in the majority of cases. Thus the "amyloid hypothesis" argues that the deposition of amyloid plaques occurs, which leads to problems with nerve cell function, which then lead to the changes in a person's cognitive abilities. Since the major and consistent component that is present in all amyloid plaques is the short amyloid beta peptide, then it follows that this peptide should be an excellent biomarker for the disease. As a biomarker, the presence or absence of this peptide in the wrong places at the wrong time is evaluated. Thus the loss of amyloid beta peptide from the cerebrospinal fluid is a useful biomarker. This loss occurs as the amyloid beta in the cerebrospinal fluid moves into the brain where it is converted into plaques. Thus another biomarker is the appearance of that amyloid beta in plaques in the brain as detected by PET (Positron Emission Tomography).

Since tau proteins make up the tangles in the Alzheimer's brain, the presence of tau protein variants is another major biomarker. (There is evidence that neurofibrillary tangles are a later event in the progression of the disease and not a cause.) Another biomarker is evidence of brain atrophy as measured using MRI (Magnetic Resonance Imaging). Yet another is the decrease in a person's cognitive function—their ability to remember and reason, for example—as revealed by various psychological tests.

It is widely believed that using two or more of the aforementioned biomarkers can serve as an indicator of the future development of Alzheimer's disease. Two questions still remain: "Are there even better biomarkers that will allow us to determine even earlier stages of Alzheimer's disease?" and "Are there biomarkers that will indicate when the disease actually starts?" These goals are shared by many doing frontline research.

The Pharmaceutical Landscape

Various pharmaceuticals have been approved worldwide to help with the neurodegenerative effects of Alzheimer's and other cognitive diseases. As with natural remedies, we need to understand why these drugs have been developed and how they work. Is there potential for a cure with any of them or are they simply a short-term but still potentially valuable stopgap? To understand the value of these drugs and to gain more insight into the cause and progression of Alzheimer's disease we will need to learn a bit about how brain cells work and how they break down in the diseased brain.

The basic truth is simple: we can't expect to find a cure for Alzheimer's disease until we understand why it occurs. We can't just randomly pull a natural or a synthesized drug out of the air and expect that it will be the wonder drug for Alzheimer's disease. We also cannot rely on unproven opinions and promotions that are presented on the Internet. Biomedical research needs to be done to understand how the disease starts and progresses and it needs to be done in a logical and sequential way though careful study. This is so results can be statistically analyzed to verify if the specific pharmaceutical actually works. How this is and should be done is detailed in later chapters. As we have seen, there is one prime candidate as a primary cause of Alzheimer's disease. It is the little peptide amyloid beta that we introduced above. These deposits are believed to alter how brain cells work by changing their cell membranes and their inner workings and may in turn cause the formation of neurofibrillary tangles. Much of today's research focuses on amyloid beta but it may not be alone in causing the symptoms of Alzheimer's disease.

The Stage is Set

The Baby Boomer cohort has had a major impact on society's progress. As more and more of this generation have entered the Alzheimer's disease-sensitive stage of life, their concern is growing. So too is their will to understand what causes Alzheimer's and to find a way to slow or stop the progress of the disease, if not prevent it in the first place. In this book, we will examine all of these issues and many more that most people have not even considered. This introductory chapter has set the stage for what follows. With the exception of topics related to care of those with Alzheimer's disease, all of the topics covered here and more will comprise the rest of the text. Most of this content will be easy to grasp by anyone but, at times, it will be necessary to delve into areas that will require a bit more effort. In such cases separate sections designated as "FYI:" are provided for those who want more details about the topics being covered. In the end a complete understanding will emerge on what we currently know and what we don't know about this devastating, life-altering disease.

Chapter 2

The Alzheimer's Epidemic by the Numbers

As discussed in Chapter 1, many consider Alzheimer's disease to be the most significant health and social crisis of this century. In other words, it is on the verge of reaching epidemic proportions that require immediate and serious attention. To paraphrase the American Heritage Dictionary, "an epidemic is any event or disease that spreads, grows or develops rapidly". Alzheimer's fits this definition because it is a worldwide disease that is spreading rapidly. Already the disease has reached close to epidemic levels — and it is projected to get much worse. As the most prevalent and one of the most severe brain diseases, the cost to individuals, families and societies everywhere on this planet will only increase over time. In this short chapter, we'll look at some specific numbers that give insight into why Alzheimer's disease is approaching epidemic proportions and, as a result, why its implications to society can't be ignored.

The Aging Crisis

The baby boom has caught up with us. As we all know, those babies have not only grown up, they have begun to senesce. In certain areas, elderly people outnumber the young by a large majority. As some would put it, we are facing a dramatic demographic upheaval that has not occurred previously in human history. While the large number of people born between 1946 and 1964 are a major part of this problem, other factors have made the situation worse. First, people are living longer. Second, fewer babies are being born due to a decrease in human fertility around the world. As a result of the large post-war baby boom, senescing populations are set to dominate demographics worldwide. While many are doing a "Chicken Little" over this, suggesting impending doom on all fronts, others suggest that if handled properly such demographic changes can often open doors to increased prosperity. Our concern here is not about the economic or social implications of this aging demographic but what it means in terms of one disease: Alzheimer's.

Why Focus on Alzheimer's Disease?

So it's a given that there are more elderly people on earth today than there ever have been in the past. As we age, we all experience a decline in memory. Often our ability to reason as quickly as we once did also takes a downhill route. Many diseases rear their ugly heads as we age. Of these diverse diseases, those affecting our ability to think, reason and remember are among the most devastating because they take away our past, our present and our future. These are the neurodegenerative diseases, of which Alzheimer's is considered to be the most common. Currently the risk of Alzheimer's dementia for someone who is 65 years of age is around 10%. When we look at the situation worldwide, the implications of this percentage are staggering. Around the globe in 2005 there were over 25 million with the disease. More to the point, these numbers are increasing with each passing year. The number of people with Alzheimer's disease globally is projected to reach almost 120 million by the middle of this century as detailed below.

The Epidemic by the Numbers

We know that Alzheimer's is not caused by a contagious agent — it is, however, directly related to aging. Since the growth rate of elderly populations is the greatest in history, then it follows that the number of cases of will also be the most that have ever been on this planet at a single time. If we look at the incidence of Alzheimer's disease in relation to age, we see that about 3% of the world population between the ages of 65 and 74 suffers from the disease. This number increases to 14% of individuals aged 75–84. For those who live to the age of 85 and beyond, the number of people with Alzheimer's disease reaches close to half (47%) of those in their age group. Some estimate that if we could live to 130 years of age, everyone would develop the disease.

In terms we can all relate to, it is estimated that a 65-year-old has a greater than 10% chance of developing Alzheimer's disease. As we throw out these numbers, it is important to note that they are all estimates. It is impossible to have exact numbers because not all cases have been verified (e.g., by post-mortem autopsy) and not all cases are reported. Also, different groups studying the relationship of age and Alzheimer's disease use different criteria to diagnose the disease. As a result they each arrive at different numbers. Looking at this in a different light, it is possible some groups overestimate numbers. Why? It is because simple but major memory decline often is listed as Alzheimer's disease when it is not. This overestimation occurs when appropriate criteria, such as the presence of Alzheimer's-specific biomarkers, are not applied. Also, in the past such evaluations were not so easily made and the attributes of true Alzheimer's disease were not fully recognized; other neurodegenerative diseases were grouped under the same large umbrella. Regardless of any inconsistencies in generating the aforementioned numbers, there is no doubt that the upcoming Alzheimer's epidemic is real and a few percentage points here or there are not going to make that epidemic any less severe.

So the numbers that are presented in this book are numbers that have been proposed by many different established and respected groups who are in the know. That said, when we toss out a number like 47%, as we did above for the incidence of Alzheimer's disease in individuals 85 and older, it is just an estimate. Just like a poll of voters about their choice of politician, it gives us some idea of the current situation but it is a number that will only be verified with time. These numbers are meant to provide some insight into specific aspects of the disease but in reality whether that number is 47, 43 or 52 is up for debate. For the most part, we'll err on the side of caution in presenting such data.

Demographics Play a Big Part

There is another side to the aging population coin. As summarized in Figure 2.1, not only is the number of elderly individuals increasing but also the number of newborns (children) is decreasing. As the following graph shows, internationally the percentage of children in the world has dropped significantly from the 1950s to today. This decrease is projected to continue at least until the middle of this century. In contrast there has been a steady increase in the number of seniors. More to the point, as seniors continue to live longer; there is a projected sharp increase in their percentage of the population as we move towards the year 2050.

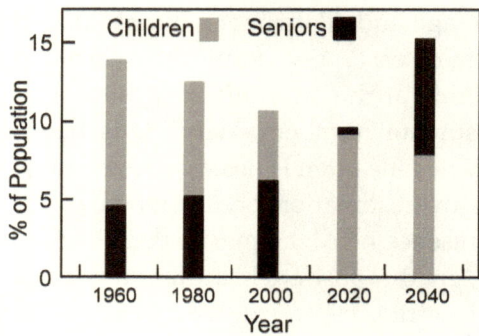

Figure 2.1. The number of children worldwide is decreasing while the number of seniors is increasing.

Because of this increased longevity, those suffering from Alzheimer's will also be around much longer than in the past, adding further to the problem. All of these factors mean the progressive and uncontrolled march towards the epidemic will continue. While estimates vary as mentioned, without question they do reflect the danger of the problems we will face. It is projected that the number of people living with dementia worldwide will almost double every 20 years. At present it is estimated that there are almost 5.5 million people with Alzheimer's disease in the US alone. This number is projected to reach almost 14 million by the year 2050. Worldwide the numbers show a similar development as reflected in the following graph (Figure 2.2).

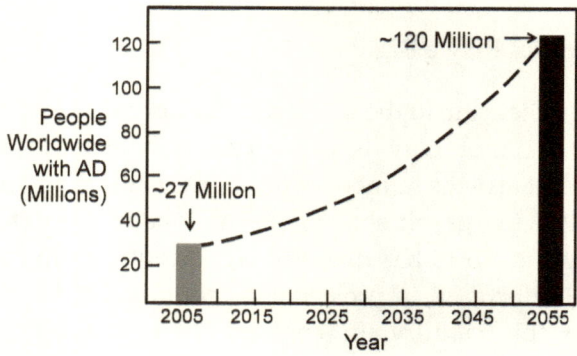

Figure 2.2. Estimates of the current and future numbers of Alzheimer's disease individuals worldwide.

In 2006, globally there were about 27 million individuals suffering from Alzheimer's disease. In keeping with the issue of getting accurate numbers as discussed above, some biomedical researchers argue this number is a low estimate. They instead suggest there are currently 50 million people worldwide suffering from the disease. This number is expected to increase almost four-and-a-half times by the middle of the century. By that time, using the conservative guesstimate, approximately 120 million people around the world will be diagnosed with Alzheimer's disease.

In Canada, the number of cases of Alzheimer's disease is projected to more than double within the next 25 years. At present over half a million Canadians suffer from Alzheimer's. More than 71,000 sufferers are younger than 65 years of age. Things don't look good for the future because currently a new case of is diagnosed every five minutes. Within 25 years or so, that number is expected to increase with a case of Alzheimer's disease being diagnosed every two minutes. Similar numbers have been reported for other countries. For example, currently in Australia there are approximately 270,000 people suffering from Alzheimer's disease. This number is projected to reach one million by 2050.

If you think about those numbers, it will immediately become clear that not only are the implications to the individual devastating but the significance to society is equally compelling. The increasing cost to healthcare alone is almost incomprehensible.

Different Countries, Different Problems

But there is another aspect to the increasing Alzheimer's epidemic. Less-well-off countries are going to pay a higher price because the number of people with the disease will be greater in those countries. Data have revealed that the development of Alzheimer's disease is directly linked to economics. Individuals from poorer countries are more likely to suffer from it than those from well-off countries. The data presented in Figure 2.4 summarize this information. As time passes, about five times more individuals will develop Alzheimer's in low- to middle-income countries compared to those in better-off countries.

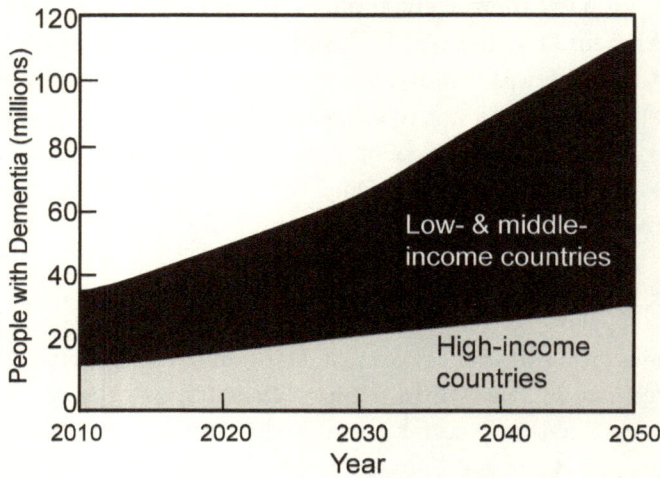

Figure 2.3. The number of individuals with
Alzheimer's disease varies based on the country's income.
(Modified from Wortman and Wimo, 2011)

What does this mean economically? Well, it's estimated that the current cost of Alzheimer's disease worldwide is over $600 billion US per year. Or, as an economist might write it: at present Alzheimer's costs us 1% of the global gross domestic product. And things are predicted to get worse. To be blunt, the cost of the disease in the US alone is projected to be in the hundreds of billions of dollars annually. Internationally the economic burden of the disease is projected at somewhere around $15 billion. Within one generation this number is expected to balloon tenfold to about $150 billion annually. While one might argue about the exact costs, there is no doubt the international economic impact of Alzheimer's will be staggering if the current situation persists. Thankfully, some countries have begun to develop action plans in the fight against the Alzheimer's epidemic.

Developing an Action Plan

While only a limited number of governments have begun to develop action plans to deal with the Alzheimer's epidemic in their country, the results of their work will help guide other governments in the future. While the action plans of those countries that have implemented them do vary, overall these plans are designed to raise awareness, improve education, improve care and garner more money for research into the disease. Research funding would go towards the search for "cures" and early diagnosis, among other things that will be detailed later. Several countries initiated Alzheimer's disease action plans during the first decade of this century. The countries showing this foresight include Australia, Denmark, England, France, Korea, the Netherlands, Norway and Sweden, among others. For example in 2008, President Sarkozy implemented the third "French Alzheimer Plan" at a cost of 1.6 billion Euros. The success of this plan was validated three years later in 2011, leading to another three-year plan being implemented. Others, such as the US and many European countries, have plans under development. In contrast, some countries such as Canada did not have a national strategy at the time this book was written. In spite of the initiatives taken by many countries, most still are ill prepared to face the reality of the Alzheimer's epidemic. Later in the book, we'll discuss what is and what can be done to reduce these numbers and costs.

Chapter 3

The Stages of Alzheimer's Disease

There are a multitude of reasons why it is critical to precisely determine the stages in the progression of Alzheimer's disease. For family members, it's essential to accept the severity of the disease so that they can make decisions about whether home care is sufficient or whether their parent or grandparent should move into a long-term care residence. For the family physician, knowledge about the status of the patient can guide him or her in suggesting the appropriate therapy. For researchers, defining the exact stage of progress of the disease is paramount. Only when the stages of Alzheimer's are well defined can effective and meaningful research be done.

Historically, much of the work to date on the disease has simply led to developing more meaningful and appropriate staging criteria. But even today, Alzheimer's research groups are fine-tuning their definitions not only of the stages but also of the specific changes that occur at each stage. As more clinical indicators of the disease are discovered, it may one day be possible to determine exactly when the disease starts. One thing we do know is that the symptoms of Alzheimer's don't appear until long after the disease has been set in motion.

The Onset and Progression of Alzheimer's Disease

Since Alzheimer's disease starts long before there are any overt symptoms, this makes the search for causes and a cure much more difficult. Figure 3.1 provides a simple summary of how the as yet undetermined initiating events precede the presymptomatic phase. As its name implies, a person shows no symptoms during the presymptomatic phase. The presymptomatic phase is followed some time later by the actual symptoms of the disease where initially observed cognitive deficiencies often progress over time. As we will learn, there are some known predictors of Alzheimer's disease. There are certain genes that are linked to the disease, for example, but the actual initiating events that drive the onset of the disease are not known.

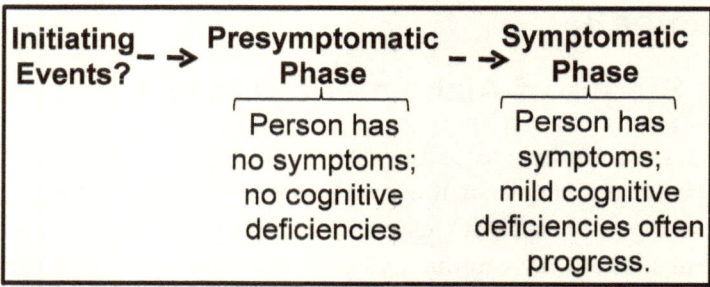

Figure 3.1. The onset and progression of Alzheimer's disease.

So, after the ground has been laid for the disease, it is followed by a long presymptomatic phase where the person appears completely normal and exhibits no cognitive deficiencies. Their memory is good, they recognize friends, family and items; they relate to the world around themselves. But during this time changes in the brain are occurring which will alter how their brain cells talk to each other. This progressive failure in brain cell communication underlies the events that will define the symptomatic phase, because without normal brain cell intercommunication, cognitive deficiencies become evident which usually can progress to greater brain malfunction.

The goal of biomedical research, and the underlying focus of this volume, is to study the progression of Alzheimer's disease from the events that initiate it through to the final changes that face individuals who develop full-blown dementia. As summarized in Figure 3.2, by asking and answering specific questions at each stage, not only can the disease be better understood but new therapies can be developed. For example, by answering the question, "How does the disease start?" researchers will ultimately answer the question of how to cure the disease. The value will be the ability to stop the disease before it starts. This, of course, is the most challenging issue. After all, how can you study something that apparently hasn't happened yet?

Knowing what happens in the presymptomatic phase prior to the onset of cognitive deficiencies will allow biomedical researchers and pharmaceutical companies to find ways to slow or prevent the progress of the disease. Of course, the problem is determining when that phase exists when there are no symptoms that are evident. This is where the role of biomarkers comes into play as detailed in Chapter 11. Dissecting out the underlying brain changes that precede the onset of mild cognitive impairment will reveal targets that can become the focus of interventions aimed at slowing or stopping the progress of the disease.

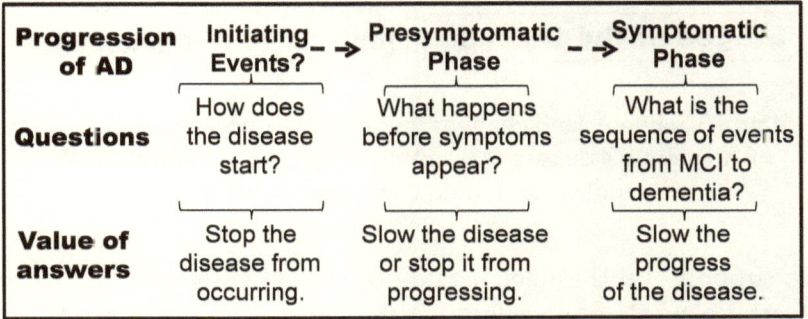

Figure 3.2. Asking and answering questions about the onset and progression of Alzheimer's disease. MCI, mild cognitive impairment.

Figure 3.3 summarizes these events, relating them to the underlying changes that are occurring in the brain and the specific stages of Alzheimer's disease. As we progress through this volume, we will learn more about each of these topics. There are known underlying brain changes that occur during Alzheimer's disease. While the actual initiating events and underlying biochemical changes are not known, during the presymptomatic phase, a substance called amyloid beta begins to accumulate (Figure 3.3, top). As mentioned in Chapter 1 and detailed in Chapter 6, amyloid beta peptides will accumulate to form amyloid plaques, one of the hallmarks of Alzheimer's disease. As this occurs the disease is progressing into the mild cognitive impairment stage of the symptomatic phase (Figure 3.3, bottom). Neurofibrillary tangles (NFTs; Chapter 7) begin to form and, coupled with the amyloid plaques, lead to progressive neurodegeneration that is linked to brain cell miscommunication and death. These events begin to transform the symptomatic phase from the mild cognitive stage to dementia as detailed later in this chapter.

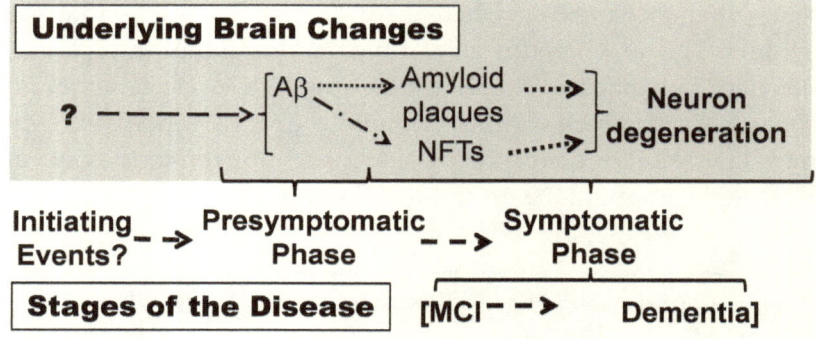

Figure 3.3. Events and changes linked to the onset and progression of Alzheimer's disease. Aβ, amyloid beta; NFTs, neurofibrillary tangles; MCI, mild cognitive impairment.

In support of this model, a study published at the end of 2012 in Lancet Neurology revealed that the appearance of amyloid beta occurs during the presymptomatic phase long before there are any overt symptoms of the disease. As the disease progresses, amyloid plaques form from accumulations of amyloid beta and other components. The accumulated evidence argues that the appearance of plaques is followed by another hallmark of Alzheimer's disease, the formation of neurofibrillary tangles (NFTs). Working on both the outside (plaques) and inside (tangles) of nerve cells, these accumulations begin to affect how nerve cells talk to each other. One might say the plaques gum up the surface of nerve cells where they contact and send messages to each other, while the tangles interfere with events inside these cells where the messages are translated and prepared to be sent on to other cells.

As the plaque and tangle populations continue to grow, nerve cell communication becomes severely compromised. The result is a progressive loss in one's ability to routinely reason fully or recall names and events, among other things. In the early symptomatic phase, this mild cognitive impairment (MCI) is often noticed by family and friends, if not the individual themselves. As the brain cells begin to deteriorate and die, MCI can progress to full-blown dementia where the person will fail to recognize or be able to relate to friends, family or the world around them.

How Does Alzheimer's Start?

What is the trigger for this devastating disease? This is the big question. It will also be the most difficult to determine. If we are ever going to prevent Alzheimer's disease from developing, we need to know when it actually starts. What is the trigger? Is it a single event or many simultaneous or temporally defined events? Is it the same for all cases or are there many initiating causes that vary from individual to individual? At the very least it will be critical to know the earliest, if not the first, changes that underlie the onset of the disease. Knowing how Alzheimer's initiates and progresses will allow biomedical scientists find ways to prevent, ameliorate and ultimately cure the disease.

The results of a diverse number of studies, meetings and conferences suggest that the underlying events of Alzheimer's disease occur long before the disease becomes evident. As summarized in the previous paragraph and indicated in Figure 3.3, the initiating events (cause or causes) that set the disease in motion are unknown. The same goes for the number of years it takes for the resulting changes to take hold. However, some advancement has recently been made in this area. The initial underlying but unknown changes in the brain are believed to be the pathophysiological underpinnings of Alzheimer's disease. They presage the clinical aspects of the disease. As mentioned, there is a long asymptomatic phase or latency period between the pathophysiological changes that occur in the brain and the clinical aspects which we see as Alzheimer's. During the latency period or presymptomatic phase, amyloid beta builds up in specific brain regions, transforming a person without symptoms into one who shows symptoms of cognitive impairment. Until very recently, scientists suggested that there was around a 10-year latency period before the cognitive effects of Alzheimer's become evident. With that timeline extended to as much as several decades, it opens up a much wider window for early diagnosis and therapeutic intervention. But what are the targets for diagnosis and intervention?

Investigations into the early events in Alzheimer's are focusing on potential biomarkers for the disease which will permit early diagnosis—the first step in being able to devise a cure in the long term and in helping the patient fight the disease in the short term. In short, current approaches to dealing with Alzheimer's disease are taking the same approach used for other diseases such as heart disease, diabetes and cancer, to name a few. For example, with heart disease, it has been shown that high LDL (low-density lipoprotein) is bad. So doctors help individuals lower the amount of this bad form of cholesterol in their blood by regulating their diet and/or prescribing medicine. If the causative agent of Alzheimer's disease, assuming there is one or at most a few, could be determined, then the quest for a cure is possible. Alzheimer's, however, may be more like cancer where multiple causes lead to multiple forms of the disease in a diversity of human tissues. Since the brain is the primary tissue of assault in the disease, then it is believed the cause or causes may be few in number but that is yet to be learned.

Thus the presymptomatic stage—the stage when no symptoms are evident—is a stage when the events of Alzheimer's disease are set in motion likely in part by the accumulation of amyloid beta. This is also called the preclinical stage because there are no symptoms that can be identified by a clinician. The changes that are occurring are happening at the cellular level, in the brain neurons where all thinking and reasoning occurs. Later we'll look at some work that is being done to identify attributes of the preclinical or presymptomatic stage that will allow for early detection and intervention. Identifying these changes could one day point to the initiating events of the disease which in turn may provide hope for a cure.

Personality Changes Can Be a Signal

As we age, significant changes in personality can be a signal that something is amiss with our brains. Or as a doctor might say, "Significant behavioral changes might be indicative of an underlying neurological disorder". Thus, changes in how a person interacts with others or behaves in the presence of others might indicate neurological changes linked to mild cognitive impairment. Similarly, when an individual starts to act differently in normal surroundings or shows deficiencies in how they deal with the activities of normal daily living, then negative neurological changes might be occurring. It is important to determine that these kinds of changes aren't due to non-neurological stresses such as family strife, breakups, financial difficulties or the multitude of daily stressors we all face in life and which affect how we behave. Having used the term "mild cognitive impairment" several times already, let's take a look at what this means because it is a key early stage in the progression of Alzheimer's disease.

As we will unravel in this volume, true Alzheimer's disease is a continuum of events rather than a stepwise process. However, we need to break it up into definable steps for simplicity and to allow us to comprehend the progress of the disease. Figure 3.4 summarizes this continuum which will be explained here, with details of each topic forthcoming throughout this book. Essentially this figure includes information that has been covered up to this point and is simply presented in a different way to show the interrelationship between the topics we've been covering and to set the stage for some future topics.

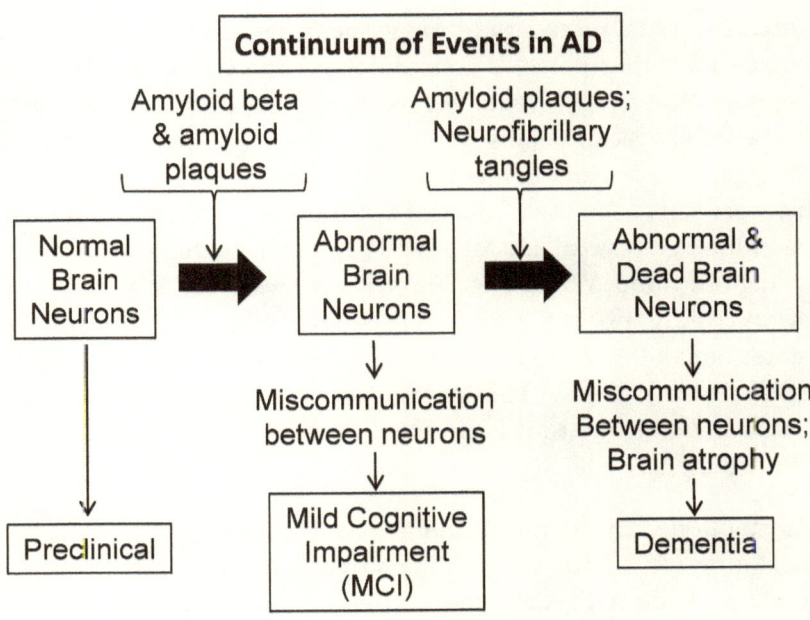

Figure 3.4. The continuum of events in Alzheimer's disease.

As mentioned above, the preclinical stage of Alzheimer's disease is when the disease is set in motion but undetectable with today's knowledge and technologies. The accumulation of amyloid beta and its coagulation or precipitation as amyloid plaques signals the early changes that are occurring in the Alzheimer's brain. These lead to miscommunication between the neurons which is manifest as the loss of memory and other attributes that define "Mild Cognitive Impairment" or MCI. As the amyloid plaques continue to accumulate, a second culprit comes into play—tangles of fine filaments in brain cells called "neurofibrillary tangles". As this is occurring, the signs and symptoms of Alzheimer's are continuing to progress, along with major changes in brain structure. These include more serious and extensive miscommunication between neurons as well as the atrophy of the brain. These changes ultimately lead to dementia. So let's begin our understanding of these events by covering mild cognitive impairment. In later chapters we'll get into the nitty-gritty of amyloid plaques (Chapter 6) and neurofibrillary tangles (Chapter 7).

MCI: Mild Cognitive Impairment

Often the initial discovery of Alzheimer's disease in an individual begins with that person's concern about their perceived loss of memory. As we age, we all get concerned about the fact we can't immediately recall details. We forget where we left our car keys or glasses. We can't remember the name of a TV show. Our memory fails us in the middle of a story when a specific fact can't be immediately recalled. All of this can make us think that we are losing our mind. When this concern becomes great enough, some of us (sadly not everyone) will go to a doctor, hoping for reassurance. In most cases, that reassurance is forthcoming. At other times it is not. This change in memory sometimes is an initial indicator that all is not well with, as Hercule Poirot put, "the little gray cells".

As mentioned in Chapter 1 and above and summarized in Figure 3.5, aging can lead to forgetfulness that doesn't progress or have anything to do with Alzheimer's disease. On the other hand, some individuals will suffer from the disease at a young age, often well below age 65. Early-onset Alzheimer's disease is discussed in various places in this book but detailed in Chapter 12 when we discuss genes linked to the disease. When Alzheimer's disease appears after age 65, it is considered to be late-onset Alzheimer's. Both early-onset and late-onset Alzheimer's disease are first evident as mild cognitive impairment. This may or may not progress. If it progresses to the severe cognitive disorder (SCD) stage, it is common for dementia to be the ultimate result. (SCD is used more commonly by those working in the field and, for simplicity, is only mentioned a few times throughout this volume.)

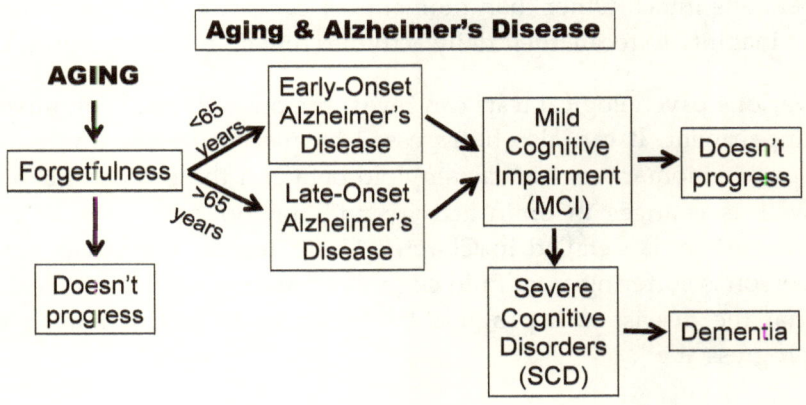

Figure 3.5. The general relationship between aging and the onset and progression of Alzheimer's disease.

So the first clinical stage for the onset of Alzheimer's is mild cognitive impairment. At this stage, close friends and family are often the first to notice changes in a person's ability to recall things or in minor changes in their ability to reason. But not all symptoms are reflected in verbal communication. Often changes in emotional behavior occur, including anxiety, anger and irrational fears such as being abandoned by a loved one. One study revealed that 80% of people with mild cognitive impairment suffer from depression, making it the most significant behavioral change associated with this stage of Alzheimer's disease. Changes in sleep patterns are also a common attribute. Of course, these are but a sampling of the changes that occur.

People suffering from Alzheimer's disease express a vast array of behavioral characteristics. Thus, clinicians and researchers need to focus on a select group of these behaviors to make their assessment of the stage that person is in. Through cognitive psychological testing, the severity of the memory impairment can be assessed. With no other explanation being present for the behavioral changes, it may be concluded that mild cognitive impairment exists. While the changes of mild cognitive impairment are of concern, people suffering from it are still able to function relatively normally because their general intellectual function remains intact. Other than moments of confusion, disorientation or inability to recall, their daily activities remain relatively normal.

Various psychological tests can reveal the onset of mild cognitive impairment. It can also be assessed by measuring the levels of specific biomarkers such as amyloid beta and the protein tau, as well as changes in brain activity and function. The subject of biomarkers is detailed in Chapter 11. To repeat, the fact that a person is suffering from mild cognitive impairment doesn't mean that the disease will progress to dementia. In fact, it may not progress at all.

Some researchers have studied the frequency of progression. As might be expected, they have found that progression is linked to age. Thus individuals over the age of 75 who had mild cognitive impairment were more than 60% likely to progress to the dementia stage. In contrast, those under 75 years of age had an over 80% chance that the disease would not progress. The severity of mild cognitive impairment was also a strong indicator of disease progression. Those who had moderate mild cognitive impairment had a 70% chance that the disease would progress compared to a chance of less than 40% for those with mild or minimal cognitive impairment. It should be noted that only a few of these studies have been done to date. Also, the number of subjects in the studies that have been carried out has been quite low. These deficiencies rule out strong statistical analyses, leaving us with only general conclusions and numbers that are less than solid. This means the numbers should not be taken strictly at face value but only used as an indicator of the general chances for disease progression from mild cognitive impairment to dementia.

Since Alzheimer's is a progressive disease, some researchers prefer to divide mild cognitive impairment into early (EMCI) and late MCI (LMCI). Just like the term SCI (severe cognitive disorders), while it is possible to define these categories with specific diagnostic procedures, it is more useful for the researcher to make such definitions than it is for us to use them as we try to understand the essence of the disease.

Attributes of Dementia: Delusions

If Alzheimer's disease does progress, it moves from these mild cognitive impairment stages to dementia. The progression of Alzheimer's disease to dementia is associated with a number of emotional changes, many of which are observed with mild cognitive impairment but now are seen with greater frequency and with heightened expression. With dementia, the person will typically experience one or more of the following: anxiety, various fears (e.g., abandonment), despair, anger and depression. They may also show compulsive behaviors and tend to suffer from hypochondria.

Delusions are also a common characteristic of Alzheimer's disease dementia. The simplest definition of delusions is that they are false beliefs, impressions or opinions. Typically the caregiver will have trouble convincing the Alzheimer's sufferer that their delusions are unfounded. Since delusions occur in about 31% of all cases, they are of serious concern to family members and caregivers. The presence of delusions in the Alzheimer's individual is often a sign of worsening behavior that likely will lead to early admission to a long-term care residence as well as increased caregiving. So there are many reasons to understand the signs and symptoms of delusions. This is typically done through the administration of psychological tests. These are carried out in conjunction with other questionnaires that assess behavior, quality of life as well as the ability to function in the real world. Questionnaires can also be given to reveal the burden that is put on caregivers who are responsible for locking after those suffering from delusional behaviors.

The accumulated research reveals that delusions arise due to the deterioration of the frontal lobe of the brain. Poor frontal lobe functioning is also linked to impaired activities in the Alzheimer's individual's daily life. CT (Computerized Tomography) scans show more lesions in frontal lobe white matter in delusional sufferers compared to normal individuals. PET (Positron Emission Tomography) studies show a reduced uptake of glucose in the frontal lobe of individuals with delusional behavior caused by Alzheimer's disease. The sugar glucose is an energy source for cells and a reduced uptake by neurons signals their decreased energy needs. This in turn indicates that these cells are less functional than normal brain cells. As if this weren't enough, delusional Alzheimer's individuals also show increased levels of amyloid plaques in their frontal lobes. These and other aspects of the Alzheimer's brain are discussed in Chapter 4 as well as elsewhere throughout the book.

With dementia, individuals progressively lose their ability to respond to the world around them. They become unable to perform the normal activities of daily life or to simply carry on a conversation. They often fail to recognize loved ones or remember who they are. This loss of cognitive awareness likely underlies many of the symptoms of the dementia stage of Alzheimer's disease where increased levels of panic and anxiety are not uncommon. Hypochondria is common in about 30% of dementia individuals. So too are increases in obsessive behavior, paranoia and depression. One study revealed that around 40% of dementia sufferers experienced one or more of these behavioral symptoms. Around 13% of individuals ultimately become antisocial while over 20% exhibit schizoid behavior. Some can become violent. Of all of these behaviors, schizoid and paranoid tendencies increase the greatest degree in the progression from MCI to dementia. Family caregivers usually are no longer able to care for the Alzheimer's sufferer by the dementia stage. Full-time care is required which often is only available in a long-term care home.

It is critical to reiterate that the severity of MCI is not a 100% predictor of progression to dementia. Not all MCI individuals will suffer from dementia. It has been estimated that about 15% of people with MCI progress to the dementia stage per year. In one study, 25% of the MCI group had not progressed to dementia even after 10 years. Currently, there is no way to determine which MCI individual will progress to full-fledged dementia.

Types of Dementia

What exactly is dementia? Dementia is an all-inclusive term that describes a variety of conditions and diseases that result from abnormal neuron function and/or death. Alzheimer's is the most common form of dementia. Your doctor might use criteria provided by the <u>Diagnostic and Statistical Manual of Mental Disorders</u> to determine if dementia exists. These criteria include a decline in one's memory along with one or more symptoms from a list.

This list includes:

- The ability to produce coherent speech;
- The ability to understand spoken language or written words;
- The ability to identify objects;
- The ability to think in an abstract way or to make sound judgements;
- The inability to function properly in daily life;
- The ability to plan and carry out complex tasks; and,
- The ability to carry out motor activities.

In addition to Alzheimer's disease, there are seven other common types of dementia that are summarized in Table 3.1.

Several dementias have Alzheimer's disease-like symptoms and this is why it is important for proper diagnostic tests to be carried out so that a disease-based therapeutic approach can be started. There are two other types of dementia listed in Table 3.1 that should be addressed as well. The extensive news coverage of "Mad Cow Disease" led many to be leery of eating beef. Mad cow disease is a prion-based disease. Prions are proteins that have misfolded. When they enter the body, prions induce proteins that are folded normally to misfold, thus interfering with normal cellular function. In the brain this leads to miscommunication between neurons and neuron death observed as holes in the brain.

A second common cause of dementia is linked to the presence of Lewy bodies in the brain. Lewy bodies are precipitates or accumulations that are rich in the protein alpha-synuclein. They cause Parkinson's disease and dementia linked to Lewy bodies. Alpha-synuclein makes up as much as 1% of the protein in brain neurons. Lewy bodies are fundamentally similar to amyloid plaques except the former consist of deposits of the protein alpha-synuclein while the latter are made up of amyloid beta. In addition, Lewy bodies form inside of neurons while amyloid plaques form outside of them. When they do appear, Lewy bodies interfere with nerve cell organization and function leading to malfunction of nerve cell communication, which underlies the dementia that is observed.

Common Types of Dementia	
Type	**Some Attributes**
Alzheimer's disease	Most common type; 60-80% of dementia cases.
Creutzfeldt-Jakob disease (CJD)	Fatal disorder that causes dementia; due to protein misfolding (e.g., prions); linked to mad cow disease.
Dementia with Lewy bodies (DLB)	Like AD but with Parkinsonian-like symptoms; involves Lewy body (alpha-synuclein) deposits.
Frontal-temporal dementia (FTD)	Progressive aphasia, Pick's disease attributes; no evident microscopic anomalies in brain; also called frontal-temporal lobar dementia (FTLD)
Mixed dementia	AD attributes plus one other such as vascular dementia or DLB; may be more common than previously thought.
Normal pressure hydrocephalus	Difficulty walking, controlling urination; due to fluid build-up in the brain.
Parkinson's disease	Results in dementia like DLB or AD; due to Lewy body (alpha-synuclein) deposits in brain.
Vascular dementia	Due to bleeding, blockage of blood vessels in the brain; initial effect: impaired judgment and ability to plan rather than memory loss.

Table 3.1. Common types of dementia.

It is important to realize that certain other conditions can result in symptoms that mimic dementia. These conditions include depression, drug use, excessive use of alcohol, side effects from medications, thyroid problems and certain vitamin deficiencies, to name the most common. When those conditions are removed or corrected then the dementia-like symptoms disappear.

The Three Stages of Dementia

While the progression of dementia varies greatly from individual to individual, the World Health Organization (WHO) and other groups define three stages. Each of these stages falls within a relatively regular timeframe and each has specific characteristics. Here we will summarize the approximate timing and specific symptoms of each stage. These stages apply not only to Alzheimer's disease, the most common cause of dementia, but also to other neurodegenerative diseases such as dementia with Lewy bodies and vascular dementia, among others.

The three stages of dementia are the following:

- **Early stage** — occurs within the first year or two;
- **Middle stage** — occurs during year two to five;
- **Late stage** — occurs from the fifth year onwards.

The following Table summarizes some of the signs and symptoms of each of the three stages of dementia (Table 3.2).

The Three Stages of Dementia		
Early Stage	**Middle Stage**	**Late Stage**
-Changes not evident; seen as normal part of aging	-Changes become clearer; more restrictive	-Total dependence; inactivity; serious memory disturbances
-Forgetful (esp. recent events)	-Very forgetful (events, names)	-Unaware of time & place
-Difficulties communicating, finding correct words	-Difficulties regarding time, date, place & events	-Can't understand events occurring around them
-Lose track of time of day, month, season, year	-Need help with personal care (dressing, toilet, washing)	-Can't recognize family, friends or familiar things
-Difficulty making decisions & handling finances	-Can't prepare meals, clean or shop	-Increased need for help with care; incontinence common
-Mood & behavior changes including depression, anxiety, anger	-Mood & behavior changes include wandering, aggression, hallucinations, disturbed sleep	-Mood & behavior changes continue to escalate with more aggression

Table 3.2. The three stages of dementia.

Thus it can be seen that early on, most people will discount many of the early-stage signs and symptoms of dementia as simply a reality of the aging process. After all, as we age we all are a bit forgetful, some more than others. We all find certain words or names elusive and may forget what day it is, especially if we are retired. It is not unusual for people at any age to show phases of anger, anxiety and depression. But when these mood changes and behaviors increase or appear in a person who normally doesn't experience them, it is time for concern. Also, when these basic signs are coupled with several other symptoms, they may be due to the early stage of dementia.

Dementia is progressive. Though it varies from person to person, the initial attributes of early-stage dementia become increasingly more pronounced as middle-stage dementia is attained. Thus early problems of forgetfulness—of words, names, time and place —are now much more common and more serious. At this stage as well, individuals are becoming less independent and much more dependent on their caregivers since help with personal care, using the washroom and dressing become a necessity. In the middle stage, serious changes in moods and behavior also become evident. While some like disturbed sleep are worrisome, others, such as wandering and hallucinations, can become dangerous.

By the late stage of dementia, the individual is fundamentally no longer able to look after him- or herself. They are no longer aware of their surroundings and issues of time and space elude them. Family and friends no longer exist for them; they are strangers, except for lapses into lucidity on rare occasion. The individual's healthcare needs are extensive and aggression, especially hitting or kicking caregivers, is not uncommon.

The transition from a cognitively functioning person to one who only exists as a former shell of themselves is one of the most disconcerting and troublesome aspects of dementia. While a major goal of Alzheimer's research is to find a cure, the search for pharmaceuticals that can slow or stop the progression of dementia is also of primary concern.

Chapter 4

The Alzheimer's Brain

Changes in the brain are the fundamental cause of Alzheimer's disease. Thus understanding the disease will require an in-depth analysis of how the normal brain changes. Since the primary concerns of Alzheimer's disease revolve around the loss of cognitive abilities—the inability to remember, reason and relate, for example—then we might simply think that only the nerve cells, or neurons, of our brain are involved. But the brain is a very complex organ made up not only of neurons but also of other cells. The functions of many of these other cells are still being revealed. Their role in Alzheimer's is also being investigated. In this chapter, some insight into the human brain will be provided as a backdrop for our progress into future chapters.

The Wiring of the Brain

The wiring of the brain is almost too complex to comprehend. The "wires" of the brain are its nerve cells, or neurons. There are approximately 100 billion neurons in the human brain. Most of these neurons form thousands of connections, or synapses, with many other neurons. These complex and multiple interconnections thus result in an essentially unquantifiable number of nerve pathways that underlie our thought processes, behaviors and memories. In a very general way, the wiring of the brain might be compared to a telephone system. Instead of dialing a specific phone number that connects you to someone so that you can interchange information, a person's sensory organs (eyes, ears, mouth, skin, etc.) send a message to the brain which listens to that message, interprets what it means and then tells the body what to do.

Like land-based telephone lines, if one critical line is cut then access to the person served by that line becomes unavailable. If a major telephone disruption occurs at a junction box, for example, then it becomes impossible to contact a large number of people served by that junction box. So we might analogize that early symptoms of Alzheimer's disease are like single cut lines that prevent direct access to other areas. However unlike a single line to one person, since there are so many brain "wires" that serve a single brain area, often that area can be reached less efficiently by other routes—just like phoning aunt Edna, who can get a message back to cousin Mohammed whose telephone line might be the one that was cut.

With further degeneration, large areas or junction boxes of the Alzheimer's brain become damaged—much like losing a trunk line in a phone network, in turn preventing access to many other areas. As we move on in this and other chapters, we will learn more about the brain wires and their interconnections. We'll learn a bit more about the "junction boxes" as well. In the end we'll have a good understanding of what happens to some of the brain regions of individuals afflicted with Alzheimer's disease—what changes are occurring and their significance to memory, cognition and basic awareness.

Why Alzheimer's Brain Cells Fail to Communicate

The brain is a diverse collection of neurons, glia and other cell types as detailed in the next chapter (Chapter 5). The changes that occur in them, particularly in the neurons, are what underlie the signs and symptoms of Alzheimer's disease. What is observed initially as significant loss of memory, disorientation and behavioral changes is a result of a loss of effective communication between the different regions of the brain that oversee these functions. In terms of brain nerve cell (neuron) function this can be the result of several events.

Brain neurons intercommunicate via synapses, small gaps between them. So a nerve impulse that is traveling along a nerve axon will arrive at a synapse. It can't jump, like an electrical spark, across this gap. Various signals called neurotransmitters, like acetylcholine and glutamate, must jump the gap to transfer the nerve impulse from one neuron to the next. Specific receptors on the dendrites of the cell body of the second neuron bind to the neurotransmitter. This binding sets up a new nerve impulse that now travels down the second nerve until it reaches another synapse. If this chain of events is affected in any way or any step in the sequence is stopped, then the affected neurons cannot function properly and normal brain function will be altered.

In addition to the alteration in neuron communication, Alzheimer's disease is also associated with the actual death of neurons. This can result from the lack of proper communication between the neurons such that a neuron becomes functionally disconnected from other neurons. In isolation, it no longer receives the signals for survival but instead turns on the death sequence—a process called apoptosis. The buildup of materials within neurons, such as the tangles that occur, can not only affect cell communication but the health of neurons leading them down the path of self-destruction.

These are but some of the changes in brain neurons that make them less than effective at doing their jobs and that make them die. In total this leads at first to the loss of normal cognitive function and may progress to full dementia with shrinkage of and holes appearing within the brain. The exact way that amyloid peptides, amyloid plaques and neurofibrillary tangles cause these changes in neurons is still under active study. We will touch on aspects of what is known as we progress in this volume.

The Alzheimer's Brain: Outside In

While a person may be diagnosed as having Alzheimer's disease, the disease can only be revealed after death. In short, only an autopsy can fully verify that a person suffered from Alzheimer's disease. This is done by looking not only at the gross morphology of the brain but also at the changes that occur in the brain cells themselves. We'll look at these brain changes, first on a macroscopic level. Then we'll look at normal and Alzheimer's brains at the microscopic level. During an autopsy, specific dramatic changes are evident in the Alzheimer's brain compared to that of a normal individual. These are summarized in Figures 4.1and 4.2. First of all, brain size overall is reduced in people with Alzheimer's disease. Second, the folds in their brains are wider, deeper and more extensive. These infoldings or depressions on the surface of the brain are called sulci (singular: sulcus). (The word sulcus is a general term referring to a deep but narrow furrow or groove.)

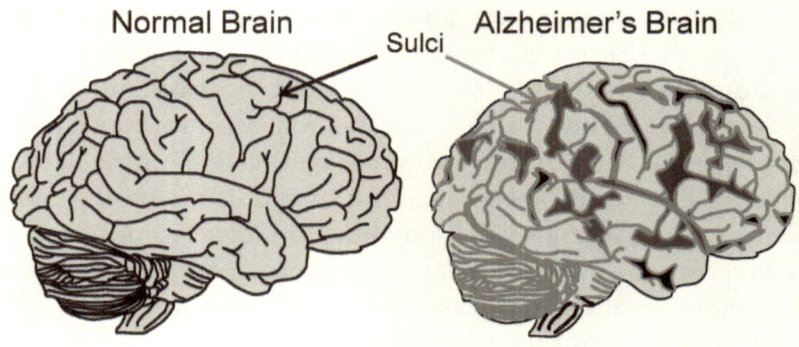

Figure 4.1. A diagrammatic representation of the surface view of a normal vs. Alzheimer's brain.

When the brain is cross-sectioned (i.e., cut open by cutting across it) to produce a brain slice, it becomes clear how far the infoldings and extensiveness of the sulci have progressed. This is shown in the diagram below (Figure 4.2), which compares the cross-section of a normal brain with that of a person with Alzheimer's. Both the marked decrease in size of the brain and the deeper sulci that characterize the disease are evident in this image.

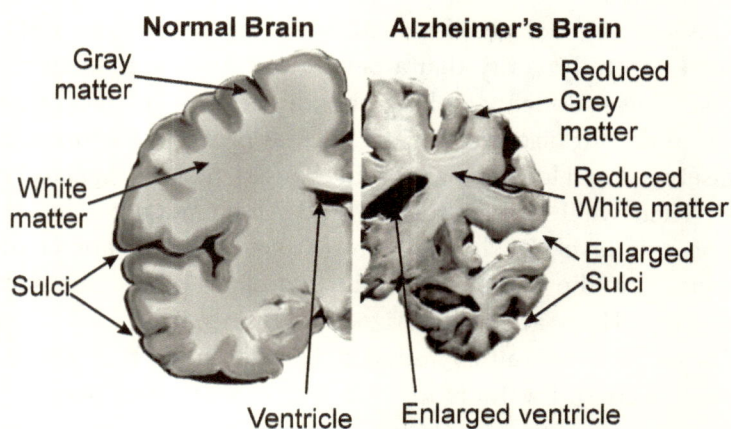

Figure 4.2. A diagrammatic cross-section image
of a normal vs. Alzheimer's brain.
(Modified from http://neurosciencenews.com/neuroscience_images/
alzheimers-disease-healthy-brain-versus-severe-public.jpg)

The sectioned Alzheimer's brain shown in Figure 4.2 also reveals how the gray matter becomes significantly reduced in the cortex of the cerebellum. The normal brain also has holes, called ventricles, which are central to its function. The word "ventricle" simply means small cavity in a body or organ. So this name is used for such brain cavities as well as those in other body organs (e.g., the heart). The ventricles of the brain are different from those seen in other organs because they are full of cerebrospinal fluid (CSF). There are four ventricles in the brain, but they become greatly enlarged in the Alzheimer's brain as indicated in Figure 4.2. This is because many millions of brain cells have died, leaving behind these large holes. To get a bit more insight, let's look at the two lateral ventricles of the brain which are used as biomarkers of Alzheimer's as revealed in an MRI scan.

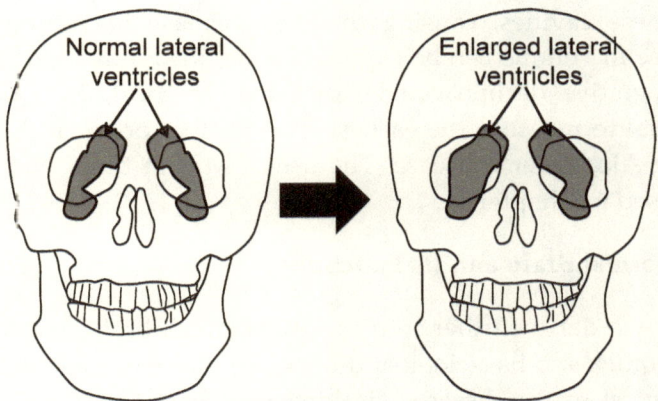

Figure 4.3. Magnetic resonance imaging (MRI) reveals the size of the lateral ventricles in the normal and Alzheimer's brain.

When you look in the mirror, if you could see through your skull and into your brain you would see these twin ventricles extending down from the center of your forehead down to behind each eye socket. The above picture shows a general diagram of these ventricles (Figure 4.3). As shown in the following figure, separate parts can be resolved as individual images by MRI, which can then be grouped to show the whole structure of the ventricles (Figure 4.4).

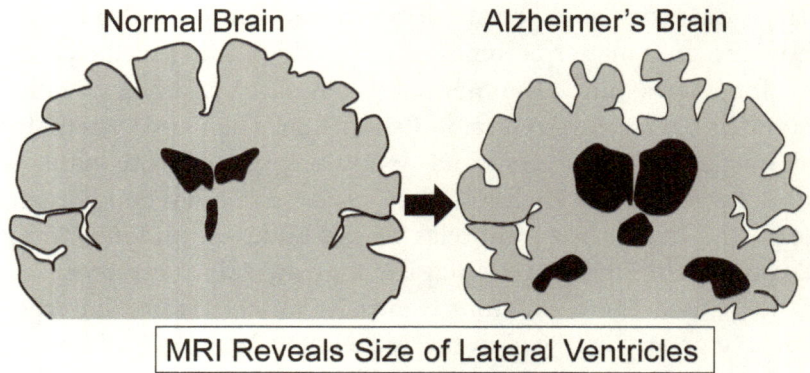

Normal Brain   Alzheimer's Brain

MRI Reveals Size of Lateral Ventricles

Figure 4.4. Brain cross-section reveals the size differences of the lateral ventricles in the normal and Alzheimer's brain.

As brain cells that surround the ventricles die they release CSF into these cavities, causing them to increase in volume. This increase in volume can be captured using MRI, often long before any cognitive decline can be detected. In short, MRI has the potential to measure the earliest changes that occur in the brain during Alzheimer's disease. The use of MRI in brain imaging is discussed in Chapter 11.

The Normal Brain and Its Functions

Before we delve further into the Alzheimer's brain, we need to take a quick and basic look at the regions of the normal brain that are central to the disease. The first goal here is not to become brain specialists—neuroscientists, neuroanatomists or even psychologists—but simply to get a basic understanding of which major brain regions become affected in Alzheimer's disease. The second goal is to gain a little bit of knowledge about the cells of the brain, especially neurons. In terms of brain regions, we will focus only on gross anatomy. In other words, we're going to look at certain brain regions overall without delving into what each sub-region does. The following simple diagram should assist in this process (Figure 4.5). The colored areas are the ones we will be concerned with. For orientation, the theoretical individual who owns this brain is currently facing to the left.

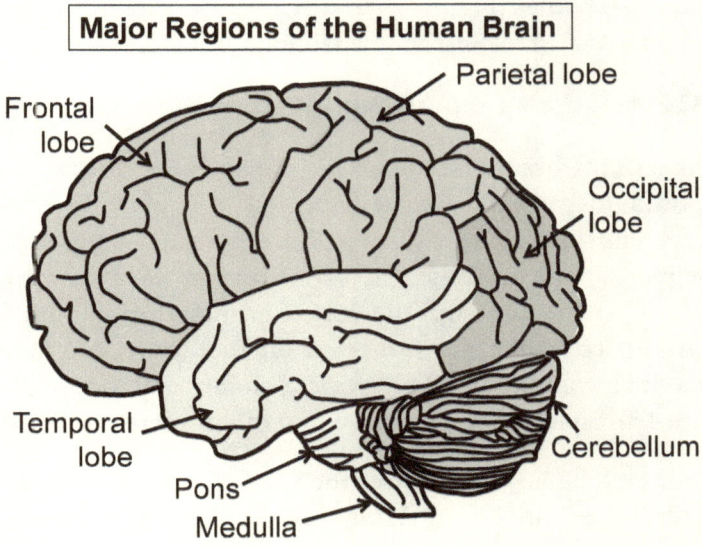

Figure 4.5. The major regions of the human cerebral cortex.

The human brain is comprised of five major parts. We are primarily concerned with the cerebrum, specifically the cerebral cortex. The cerebral cortex overlies the rest of the cerebrum and most of the other brain regions. It is the area of gray matter shown in Figure 4.2 that is involved in consciousness, language, memory, thought and awareness of our surroundings. In spite of these important roles it is only between two and four millimeters thick but there is still lots of room for billions of neurons!

We also need to understand one other aspect of neurobiology: the difference between gray matter and white matter. These are indicated in figure 4.2. This distinction mainly has to do with the organization of nerve cells in the brain. A nerve cell or neuron has a big mass of cytoplasm called the cell body which is gray in color. From this cell body, smaller projections called dendrites extend out to make contact with other nerves. Also extending from each cell body are one or more long axons. The nerve axons appear white because they are coated with an electrical insulator, a whitish myelin sheath. So the gray matter (region of neuron cell bodies) is evident in the outer layers of the brain while the white matter is more internal, showing where the axons extend away from the cell bodies (Figure 4.2). Now, let's see what this means to us in terms of normal and abnormal brain function.

The Cerebral Cortex and Alzheimer's Disease

The area of the brain that makes us human is the cerebral cortex. It is used to calculate, create, imagine and plan. It is also a primary site for changes during the onset and progression of Alzheimer's, which gives you some further idea of why the disease is so devastating. The cortex is made up of four large regions or lobes that are indicated on the above diagram: the frontal lobe, temporal lobes, parietal lobes and occipital lobe (Figure 4.5). So let's look at some of the things these regions do.

The frontal lobe lies right above the face. It is involved primarily in controlling initiative, insight, organization, personality and planning. On either side of the brain, at one's temples, reside the temporal lobes. The temporal lobes are important in the early and progressive stages of Alzheimer's disease. The temporal lobes control memory. They are also involved in speaking and understanding the words of others. A third critical role is that of processing and interpreting sounds. The parietal lobes are located at the top and back of the head. The parietal lobes play a role in sensory functions because they integrate input from the eyes and ears. They also mediate the sense of touch. If that weren't enough, they play a central role in the recognition and use of numbers. The last region of the cortex is the occipital lobe. It resides at the very back of the head just above the neck where it functions primarily in vision.

* * *

Interesting Factoid: While the brain only makes up about 2% of body mass it consumes 20% of the oxygen used by the body. The vast majority of energy is used by the neurons, so oxidative stress can play a key role in the pathogenesis of mental disorders.

* * *

We also need to consider a region of the brain that is not part of the cortex. It is the cerebellum. Lying below the occipital lobe, it is important in the late stages of Alzheimer's disease because it controls movement. In addition to controlling motor functions, the cerebellum also has some function in language and attention. Finally, this tri-lobed structure also functions in fear and pleasure to some degree.

Having said all this, it is important to emphasize that we are taking a very basic view of brain function. First, we should remember that the brain has two sides or hemispheres, right and left, each of which has distinct side-related functions. These sides as well as other brain regions need to be in constant communication. To make an analogy, the various regions of the brain are not distinct unconnected offices in a business where different events take place without consideration for what's going on in the other offices. The different regions of the brain are interconnected and work as a team to ensure that a person functions normally. So when one part of the brain begins to fail it can also have significant, life-altering effects on other brain regions and, hence, other human functions.

Alzheimer's Disease Sequentially Affects Brain Functions

Since we are not biomedical scientists or neuroanatomists, we don't need to know the fine details of how Alzheimer's progression impacts the brain. The goal here is to understand that Alzheimer's disease doesn't just randomly hit various regions of the brain. Instead, it typically follows a routine pathway of progression. Generally it is recognized that the spread of the disease in the brain occurs via known neuroanatomical pathways. That said, using the above information and the following simple diagram, we can summarize the sequence of events that commonly occur in the Alzheimer's brain (Figure 4.6).

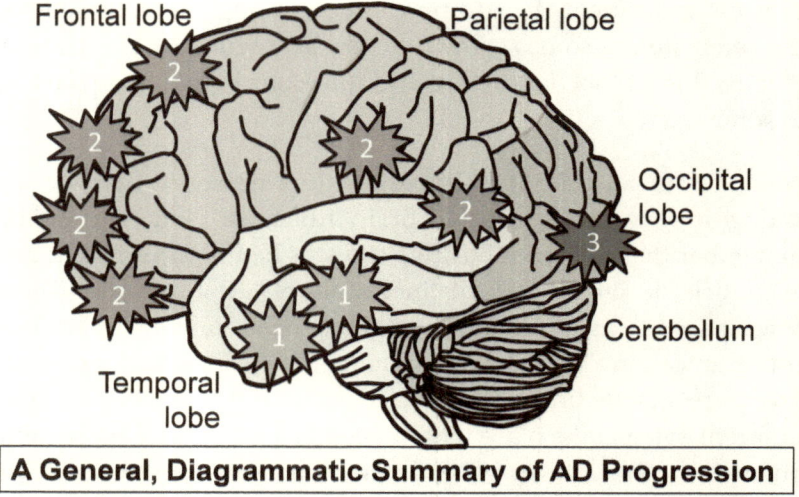

Figure 4.6. A general summary of the regions that are progressively affected in the Alzheimer's brain over time.

In the early stages of Alzheimer's disease, the first evident changes in brain structure and function occur in the cortex of the temporal lobe (1 in Figure 4.6). Plaques and tangles begin to appear that affect learning and memory as well as thinking and planning. This is followed by diffuse spreading of plaques and tangles across the cortex of the frontal lobe (2 in diagram) as we enter mild to moderate stages of Alzheimer's disease. This impacts one's ability to speak and also understand what others are saying. It also affects one's perception of themselves in relation to the world around them. At advanced stages, accumulations of plaques and tangles occur in the cortex of the occipital lobe (3 in diagram) as well as other areas. Now in the severe stages of Alzheimer's, the individual will no longer be able to care for himself or herself. They will no longer be able to communicate effectively and will no longer recognize family members or loved ones. In the following chapter we'll look at the cells that make up the brain and some of the changes that occur in them during the onset and progression of Alzheimer's disease.

Chapter 5

Brain Cells, Plaques and Tangles

While we typically think of the brain as being made up of nerve cells, they are not the only cell type that is present. To once again paraphrase Hercule Poirot, the famous Belgian detective, "We use the little gray cells to solve mysteries." Clearly our brains are referred to as gray matter because the cell body of nerve cells, which contains the nucleus and most of the cell cytoplasm, appears gray. But there is more to the brain than this. In addition to neurons, there are numerous other cell types. We'll look at just a few of these including microglia, astrocytes, ependymal cells and oligodendrocytes. As we will see later, some of these cells have also been linked to removing some of the peptides linked to Alzheimer's disease.

So let's look at the four non-nerve cell types we've chosen before we go into some depth on brain neurons.

Microglia

Astrocytes, microglia and ependymal cells are types of glia. The name glia comes from the Greek word for glue but they are more than that. Glia are present in the same number as neurons in the brain.

Microglia are considered to be brain macrophages. Macrophages are white blood cells which are key players in the immune system of our bodies. Their fundamental role is to ingest harmful cells and materials (a process called phagocytosis) to fight diseases and infections. In the brain, microglia serve as the immune system. While the blood–brain barrier keeps out most noxious substances and foreign cells, sometimes this barrier isn't sufficient. When infections occur, microglia fight off the dangerous agents that could cause inflammation or other brain damage.

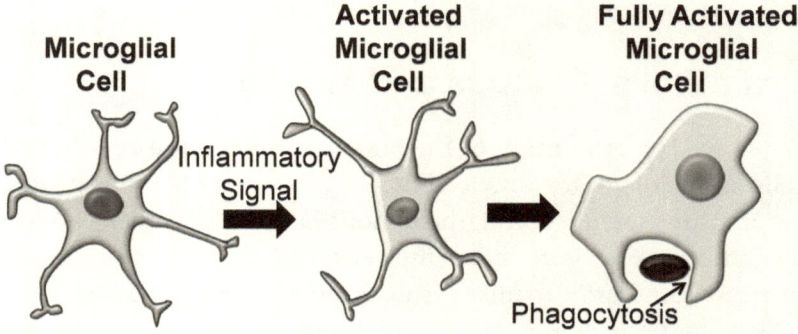

Figure 5.1. Inactivated and inflammation-activated brain microglia.

Figure 5.1 shows the structure of a microglial cell. When damage occurs to the brain or when an infection occurs, inflammatory signals are received by the microglia. This causes them to change. In response, they become activated and then differentiate into fully activated microglial cells. Like macrophages in the blood, the fully activated microglia can engulf bacteria and cell debris as well as other noxious agents.

Astrocytes

As their name implies, astrocytes are star-shaped cells (Figure 5.2, left panel). There are actually three types of astrocytes. They are a subtype of glial cell, so they are also known as astroglia. However, they show a different pattern of distribution in the brain from microglia. Astrocytes are found in the brain and spinal cord where they serve a diverse number of functions including nervous system repair, modulating nerve cell function as well as regulating components present outside of the brain cells. They also function in the blood–brain barrier. Of importance here is their role in supporting and communicating with nerve cells.

Astrocytes   GFAP

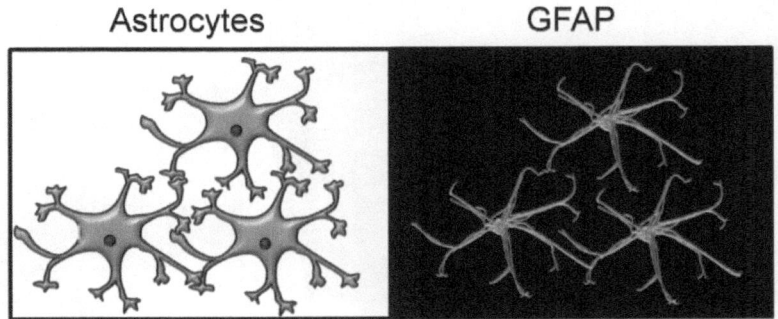

Figure 5.2. The structure of astrocytes and the organization
of GFAP within their cytoplasm.

Astrocytes are easily identified because they produce a unique protein called glial fibrillary protein or GFAP. GFAP forms part of the cytoskeleton of astrocytes (Figure 5.2, right panel). Like our skeleton, the cytoskeleton of cells is important in maintaining their shape and regulating their movement. In Chapter 7 we'll mention other cytoskeletal components like actin and microtubules which are present in all cells in our bodies. GFAP is part of a third group of cytoskeletal components called intermediate filaments. While intermediate filaments are a common cell component, GFAP is only found in astrocytes. The diagram shows typical astrocytes and how GFAP is organized within them.

Ependymal Cells

The ependymal cells line up to form a thin layer or sheet of cells called an epithelium. The thin epithelium of ependymal cells lines the ventricles of the brain. An epithelial layer of ependymal cells also lines the central canal of the spinal cord. The brain ventricles and spinal cord central canal are filled with cerebrospinal fluid (CSF). Ependymal cells are another form of glial cell that takes up, releases and moves CSF (Figure 5.3). Like epithelial cells of the human intestine, the ependymal cell surface is infolded as multiple microvilli as shown in the figure.

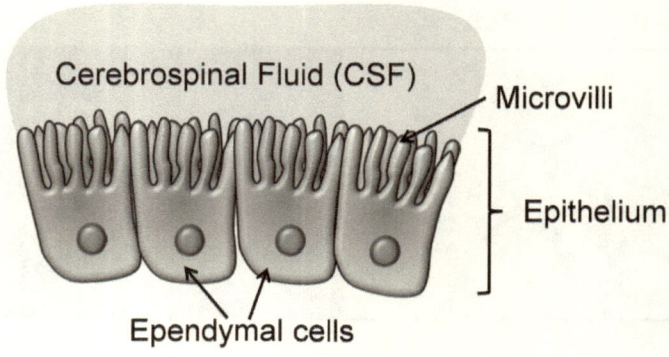

Figure 5.3. A row of ependymal cells.

Microvilli increase the surface area of cells that are active in absorbing materials. Also present on the surface of the ependymal cells are tiny hair-like projections called cilia. Cilia are like short flagella, best known as the long tail that drives sperm cell movement. Groups of cilia work as a team keeping fluid moving in various tissues and organs in our bodies. In the central nervous system, they keep cerebrospinal fluid flowing. In Alzheimer's disease, the ependymal cells secrete excess cerebrospinal fluid that will fill the enlarging brain ventricles that characterize the disease as discussed in the previous chapter (Figures 4.3, 4.4).

Oligodendrocytes

Oligodendrocytes function to insulate neurons in the central nervous system. They form myelin (white matter) and other components that surround the axon of nerve cells. Myelin allows the electrical signal in nerves to move efficiently from one end of the cell to the other. Thus, by making this special insulation, oligodendrocytes make nerve conduction in the brain and spinal cord much more efficient (Figure 5.4). (Schwann cells do the same thing for nerves outside of the brain and spinal cord, in the peripheral nervous system.) Oligodendrocytes also provide a support function for central nervous system neurons.

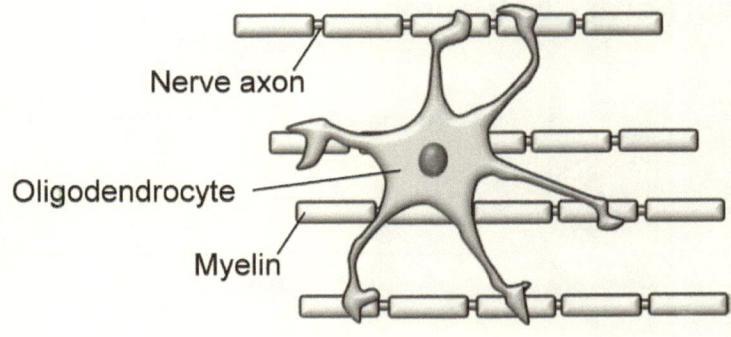

Figure 5.4. An oligodendrocyte.

Oligodendrocytes can form myelin around many neurons at the same time, unlike Schwann cells which only associate with a single neuron. The loss of myelin (demyelination) due to damaged or altered oligodendrocytes is an underlying symptom of multiple sclerosis.

Some of the aforementioned cell types will be touched upon again because more and more insight is being gained into their roles in Alzheimer's disease. However, as we progress, our primary interest will be on normal brain neurons and the changes in them that are associated with Alzheimer's. So let's take a look at what a nerve cell is and how it works. As we move ahead, we'll learn some new attributes of nerve cells and how they are being targeted in the search for a cure for Alzheimer's.

Nerve Cells

Nerve cells are also called neurons. They consist of a cell body with multiple projecting dendrites and one or more axons (Figure 5.5).

Brain Nerve Cell (Neuron)

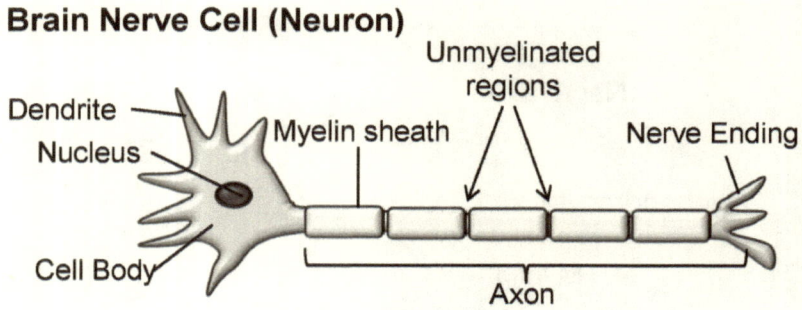

Figure 5.5. The structure of a brain nerve cell or neuron.

Nerves can either be myelinated or unmyelinated (Figure 5.6). The myelin sheath acts to insulate the neuron, preventing leakage of ions and enhancing the rate of nerve transmission. But myelin is not a continuous sheath like the coating that surrounds electrical wires in our house. There are spaces between the regions of myelin.

In myelinated neurons, rather than the nerve impulse flowing like electrons in our house wiring, the nerve impulse jumps along the axon of the nerve cell. This "jumping" over the myelinated to unmyelinated region greatly speeds up nerve cell transmission. In the brain, the white matter is the region where myelinated axons predominate while the gray matter is the primary site of nerve cell bodies.

Brain Neurons Communicate via Neurotransmitters

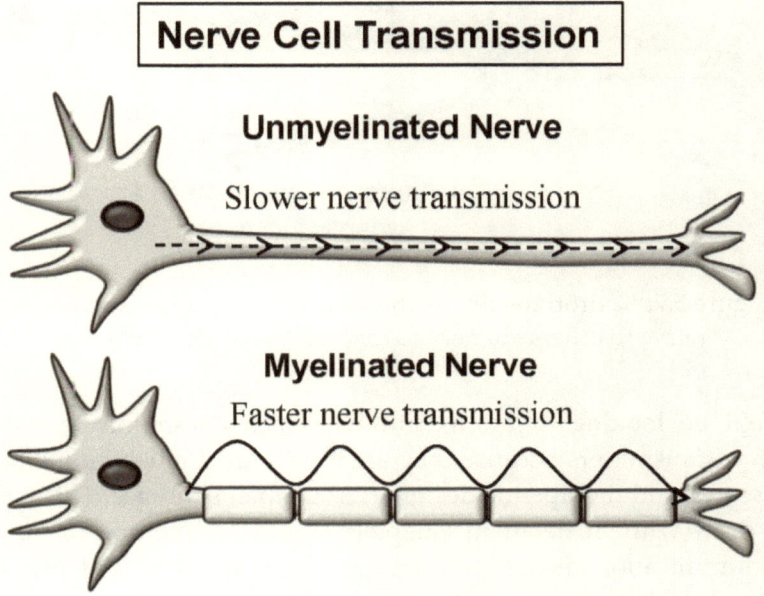

Figure 5.6. A comparison of nerve transmission in a non-myelinated versus a myelinated neuron.

There are many different types of neurons in the body but for our purposes we'll focus on those that look like our diagrammed myelinated nerve cell because these predominate in the brain. While we're looking at neurons with a single axon, most neurons have more than one while many have large numbers of axons. In the end, all of these types function the same way. The only difference is the number of interconnections with other brain neurons that are possible. Neurons interconnect by the nerve endings of one associating with the dendrites of the next.

Brain Neurons Use Neurotransmitters

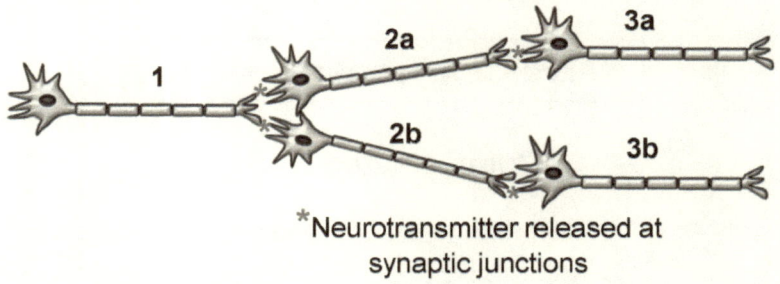

*Neurotransmitter released at
synaptic junctions

Figure 5.7. Neurotransmitters transfer the nerve impulse from one
nerve to others via nerve synapses (synaptic junctions).

We'll be looking at brain neurons which communicate using neurotransmitters because they are the focus of much biomedical research and therapeutic design in Alzheimer's disease. This topic is dealt with in detail in Chapters 9 and 10. Neurotransmitter communication means one neuron stimulates the next one by releasing chemicals from the nerve endings. After all, neurons in the brain are not directly connected. There is a space (the synaptic cleft) between them. The nerve impulse traveling down one nerve cell can't jump this gap directly. Instead, this impulse causes the release of chemicals at the gap (or nerve synapse). The neurotransmitter diffuses across the synapse and then stimulates the next neuron. This sets up an electrical impulse in the neuron that travels down its axon to again release a chemical from its nerve endings. A simple example involving several neurons is shown in Figure 5.7.

Without getting too technical, the chemicals (neurotransmitters) that are released can have a positive impact (i.e., stimulate the next nerve) or negative impact (inhibit the next nerve). All of the multitudes of neuronal interconnections with all their diverse stimulatory and inhibitory effects define how our brain remembers, responds to information and modifies our behaviors. Thus anything that affects nerve cell structure or function will affect how the brain works. And that's what happens with Alzheimer's disease.

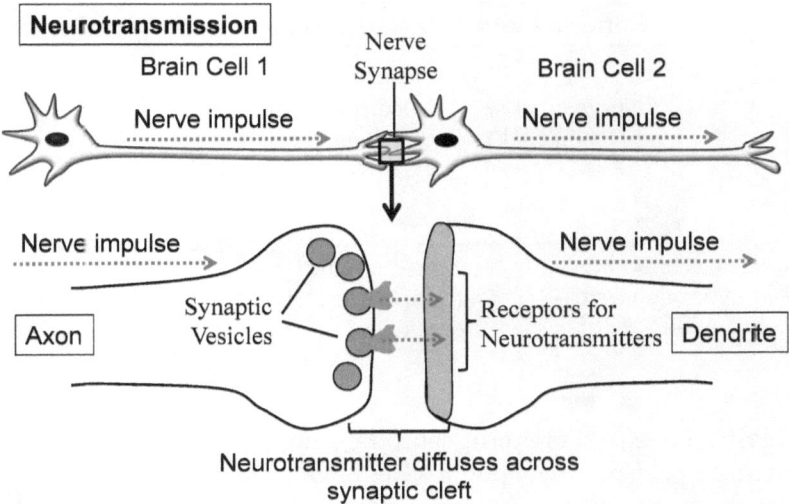

Figure 5.8. Neurotransmitters are used for communication between neurons in the brain.

As shown in Figure 5.8, a space or nerve synapse exists between brain neurons (Brain Cell 1 and Brain Cell 2). The electrical impulse can't jump this gap. Instead, the impulse causes synaptic vesicles in the first neuron to release their contents into the synaptic cleft. Synaptic vesicles are tiny bags full of neurotransmitters and other substances. The contents of synaptic vesicles are complex and nerve cell specific. They include neurotransmitters such as acetylcholine and glutamate that are covered as pharmaceutical targets in Chapters 9 and 10, respectively.

Now that we've looked at nerve structure and neurotransmitter release, let's go over the complete sequence of what happens during neurotransmission. Figure 5.9 summarizes the neurotransmitter events at a general synapse. The neurotransmitters in synaptic vesicles are released in response to an incoming nerve impulse in Brain Cell 1. The released neurotransmitter diffuses across the synaptic cleft and binds to its receptor, setting up the next nerve impulse in Brain Cell 2. Other molecules are also released into the synapse. Some of these are enzymes that will digest the neurotransmitter as a way of controlling how the neurotransmitter works and making sure it doesn't stimulate the next nerve too much or for too long.

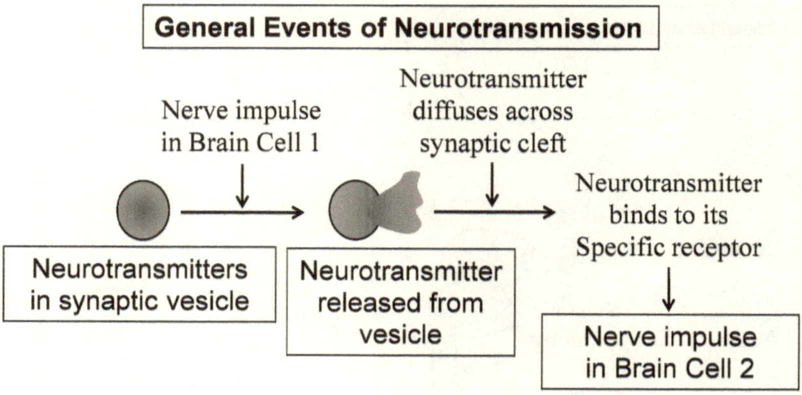

General Events of Neurotransmission

Nerve impulse
in Brain Cell 1

Neurotransmitter
diffuses across
synaptic cleft

Neurotransmitter
binds to its
Specific receptor

Neurotransmitters
in synaptic vesicle

Neurotransmitter
released from
vesicle

Nerve impulse
in Brain Cell 2

Figure 5.9. General events of neurotransmission. Neurotransmitters that are present in synaptic vesicles are released from the ends of one neuron in response to a nerve impulse. They then diffuse across the synapse where they bind to their specific receptor, setting up a nerve impulse in the next neuron.

Since brain cells communicate via neurotransmitters and since many Alzheimer's therapies are based on controlling them, let's summarize what we've covered by listing the events in sequence. The numbered sequence of events is shown in Figure 5.10 and listed in point form below.

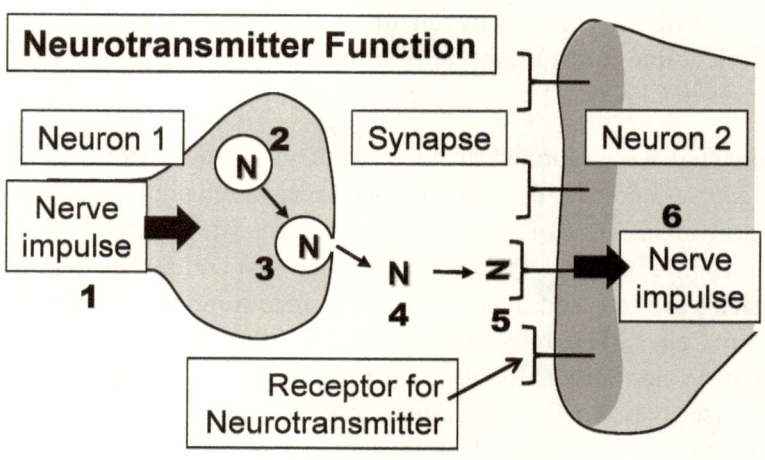

Figure 5.10. Neurotransmitter function in brain neurons.

A nerve impulse (1) travelling down the first neuron (Neuron 1) stimulates vesicles (2) containing neurotransmitter (N) to move to the neuron membrane (3) and release the neurotransmitter into the synapse. The released (4) neurotransmitter diffuses across the synapse. At the second neuron (Neuron 2) the neurotransmitter (5) binds to its receptor. This sets up a nerve impulse (6) in the second neuron.

Plaques and Tangles

As mentioned and as we will detail in Chapters 6 and 7, plaques and tangles are the hallmarks of Alzheimer's disease. Amyloid plaques form outside of nerve cells in the extracellular environment (Figure 5.11).

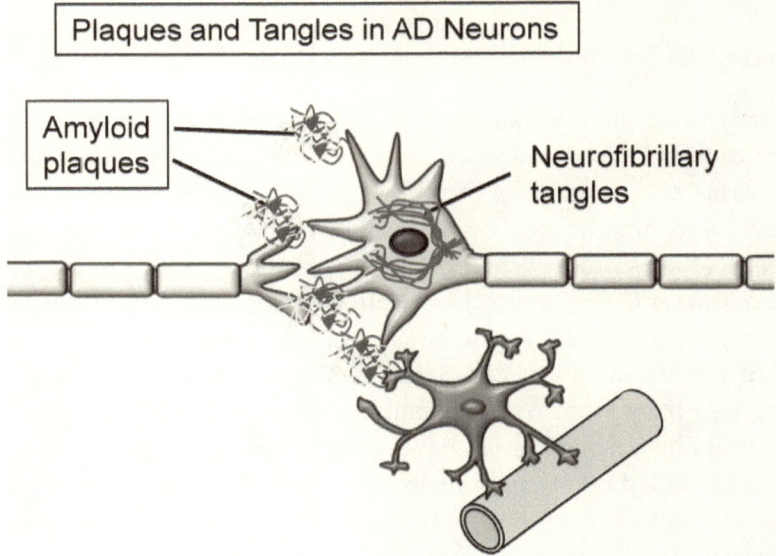

Figure 5.11. Plaques and tangles in the Alzheimer's disease brain.

By gumming up the outside of cells, including synapses, amyloid plaques dramatically affect how nerve cells talk to each other and to other brain cell types. The figure above shows how amyloid plaques can associate and interfere with nerve synapses and with glial cells. Amyloid plaques also interfere with the surfaces of neurons, which has many other effects not only on nerve cell communication but on the cells' ability to survive. On the other hand, neurofibrillary tangles form inside of nerve cells where they interfere with how the nerve cell translates incoming messages and, likely, neurotransmission (Figure 5.10). That said, exactly how plaques and tangles do their dastardly deeds is still under intense investigation.

Later we'll learn about the role of amyloid plaques and neurofibrillary tangles in Alzheimer's disease as well as what they are made of and how they are being studied in the quest for diagnosis, prevention and a cure. While plaques and tangles are believed to be a primary cause of the loss of nerve cell communication that underlies the neurodegenerative aspects of Alzheimer's, they are also implicated in the death of brain cells that causes a decrease in brain size and increased "holes" in the brain.

Brain Cell Death during Alzheimer's Disease

It may be difficult to fathom, but the fundamental events that kill brain cells in Alzheimer's disease and other neurodegenerative diseases are the same as those that are essential for normal brain development. The process is known as controlled or regulated cell death. Its more formal name is apoptosis. During embryonic development, the controlled death of cells is important in the formation not only of the brain but also of other organs. For example, the death of cells leads to the formation of the fingers and toes from what was originally a paddle-shaped mass of cells. During the formation of the ovaries, millions of potential egg cells are killed off for reasons that are yet fully understood. So not all cell death is bad; it is only bad when it occurs in the wrong place at the wrong time—as it does in Alzheimer's disease.

The death of brain cells occurs early in the disease. It contributes to the cognitive impairment that is observed. In addition to brain cell miscommunication, the loss of neurons also affects memory, logic and reasoning. It ultimately is reflected in the inability of a person with Alzheimer's to recognize the world around them and remember anything at all. In addition to these symptomatic effects, the death of neurons also becomes evident as the dramatic changes that occur in the brain itself. It is responsible in part for the shrinkage of the brain and it underlies the increase in size of the sulci and ventricles. So if we could stop brain cell death, we could at the very least stop the inexorable progression of the disease.

Chapter 6

What Are Amyloid Plaques?

There is no doubt that the amyloid hypothesis dominates the field of Alzheimer's research. This hypothesis argues that the appearance of amyloid beta in the brain and its coalescence into amyloid plaques is a central pathomechanism leading to Alzheimer's disease. Amyloid plaques continue to be a defining attribute of Alzheimer's disease. In fact, amyloid plaques and neurofibrillary tangles are widely and historically considered to be the primary causes of brain cell dysfunction and death.

What is most amazing is that over 100 years ago Dr. Alzheimer himself stated that senile plaques, tangles and the loss of brain cells were the hallmarks of the senile dementia disease that now bears his name. These three telltale signs—plaques, tangles and brain cell death—still serve to define the disease today. Here we will look a bit more into the structure of amyloid plaques. In the next chapter (Chapter 7) we will examine neurofibrillary tangles and how they are formed. The death of brain cells appears to be caused, at least in part, by the accumulation of these two components and will be discussed as well.

After introducing the formation of amyloid plaques and examining some of the diverse constituents present in these plaques we will then detail what is known about how amyloid plaque formation begins. In Chapter 8 we will detail research being done to slow or stop plaque formation.

The Detection of Amyloid Plaques

Amyloid plaques are generally considered to be insoluble clumps of amyloid beta peptides that accumulate outside of brain cells. They can't be seen or studied until an autopsy has been performed. If they are present in a person's brain then they can easily be detected after thin sections of the brain are taken and stained with appropriate chemicals as summarized in Figure 6.1.

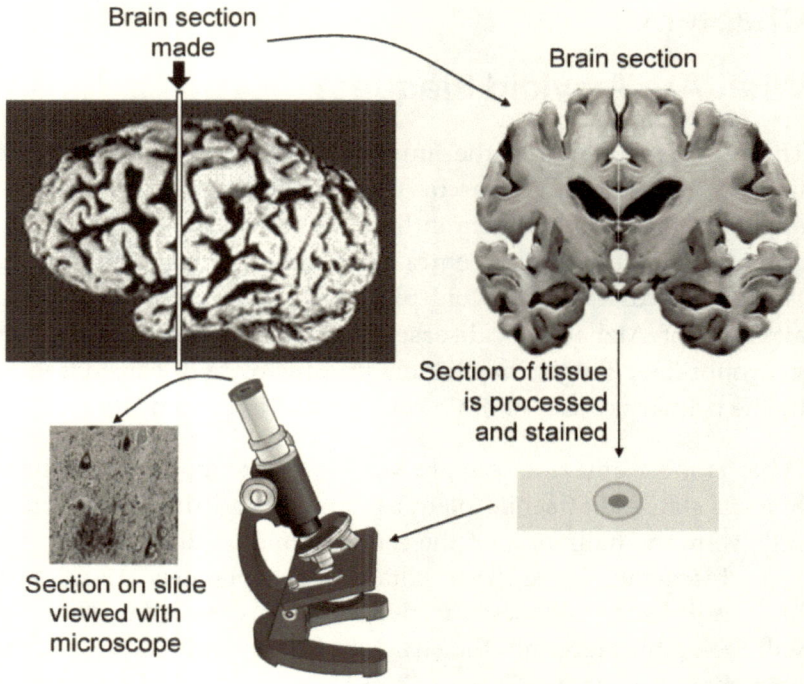

Figure 6.1. Summary of steps involved in making a slide of brain tissue to evaluate the presence of plaques.

Two different histological sections from Alzheimer's brains are shown in Figure 6.2. On the left, the brain section has been stained with the classic hematoxylin and eosin (H&E) stain which gives a pinkish background with amyloid deposits showing as darker pink/reddish masses outside of the brain cells. When brain sections are stained with a silver stain, the plaques appear as diffuse brownish masses as seen in the image on the right side of Figure 6.2. Note the darker brown cells: this stain also picks up neurofibrillary tangles inside of Alzheimer's neurons as discussed in the next chapter.

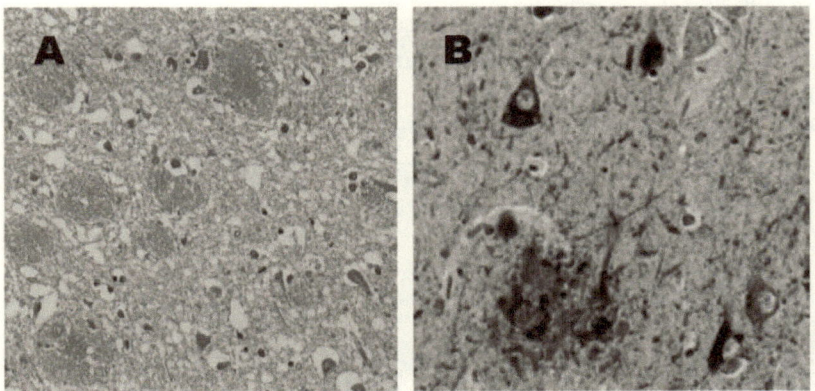

Figure 6.2. Amyloid plaques in the human brain.
A. Hematoxylin–eosin stain. B. Silver stain.

The Structure of Amyloid Plaques

If we are ever going to understand how Alzheimer's disease progresses, find a cure or prevent the disease, it is essential to understand the structure of amyloid plaques. It is also critical to understand how they first form and develop. The reality is, amyloid plaques are more than just clumps of the amyloid beta peptide. The simple sequence of diagrams shown in Figure 6.3 and Figure 6.4 should help with understanding how plaques form and change.

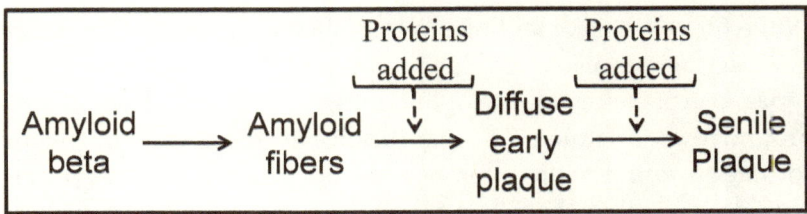

Figure 6.3. The sequence of events in the transformation of amyloid beta peptides into senile plaques.

Amyloid plaques form in a very specific way that involves a known series of steps. First, the amyloid beta peptides that are clipped off brain cells become joined together outside those cells in such a way as to form long, relatively straight amyloid fibrils or fibers. These fibers then clump together and associate with many other proteins as they form discrete plaques. The plaques that first appear are called "diffuse early plaques" (Figure 6.3, 6.4). As these plaques accumulate more amyloid fibrils and more non-amyloid proteins, they are transformed into "senile plaques". The other non-myeloid proteins that are present within these plaques are discussed below.

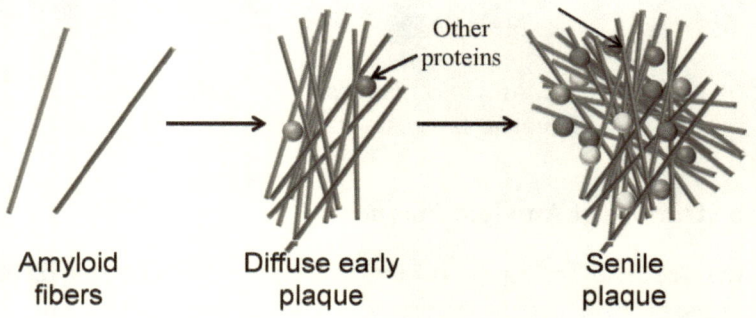

Amyloid fibers   Diffuse early plaque   Other proteins   Senile plaque

Figure 6.4. A diagrammatic representation of the transformation of amyloid fibers into a diffuse early plaque and then into a senile plaque by the progressive accumulation of amyloid fibers and other non-amyloid proteins.

Glia and Amyloid Plaques

While the protein content of amyloid plaques has been of primary interest, there is also a cellular component. Two specific brain cell types, astrocytes and microglial cells, appear and form a halo around these plaques. The significance of these cells in plaque formation and function remains to be detailed. However few would doubt that there is a significant interplay between these microglial cells, the plaques themselves and the neurons that are affected by them. First of all, the astrocytes and microglia could alter the structure of the plaques. They could also be involved in amyloid turnover by removing excess amyloid peptides and fibers. In addition, the plaques themselves may in turn affect the behavior of these cells. The structure and function of astrocytes and microglial cells were detailed in the previous chapter (Chapter 5).

* * *

FYI: Clarification of Terms Used

While our goal is to clarify things as simply as possible and be consistent with our usage of terms, it is also important to understand the formal terminology and abbreviations that are used. In this book we will be focussing on amyloid plaques that are formed from amyloid beta peptides. However while the term "amyloid plaque" is commonly used when we discuss Alzheimer's disease, amyloid deposits are much more common than we might think. The word "amyloid" is actually a much more general term that refers to deposits or accumulations of a diversity of insoluble proteins. These deposits are caused by the misfolding of proteins which then makes that protein insoluble. Proteins typically have specific shapes that not only keep them in solution but are essential for their function. When this shape is changed or misfolded, they can precipitate out of solution, forming harmful deposits in tissues and organs. Well over a dozen proteins that become insoluble due to misfolding have been identified.

Typically the deposits of amyloid proteins form outside of cells. In addition to Alzheimer's which is characterized by amyloid beta, amyloid deposits are found in many other diseases. In diabetes mellitus 2, deposits of a protein called amylin are found in the pancreas. Similar to amyloid beta, the proteins in the plaques become strung together and combined to form threadlike fibers, filaments or fibrils. To reiterate, the difference is that plaques that characterize Alzheimer's disease are primarily made of amyloid beta while other types of amyloid deposits consist of other major proteins.

* * *

Some Proteins Found in Amyloid Plaques

Not only do amyloid plaques contain a diversity of components but there is also a lot of variability in both plaque structure and content. So while characterizing the makeup of amyloid plaques has led to the identification of some consistent components, the importance of the other less consistent components remains elusive. Although the comparison may not be 100% correct, think of amyloid plaques as a sticky substance—like a drop of syrup on a countertop or your clothes—where anything that touches it can stick, making the original spot larger and more complex. Whether this is true for amyloid plaques is a question that is still under analysis. And, unlike a sticky spot, certain constituents are present in essentially all amyloid plaques and therefore are deserving of consideration as Alzheimer's-specific components. So let's take a closer look at some of the protein constituents that have gained prominence in the eyes of researchers.

It turns out that dozens of proteins are consistently found in amyloid plaques. It is critical for researchers to understand what proteins are associated with Alzheimer's plaques because these can provide insight not only into how plaques form but also why they form. These proteins could also give insight into how to prevent or slow plaque formation. Let's look at a few of those proteins that are of current interest to biomedical researchers.

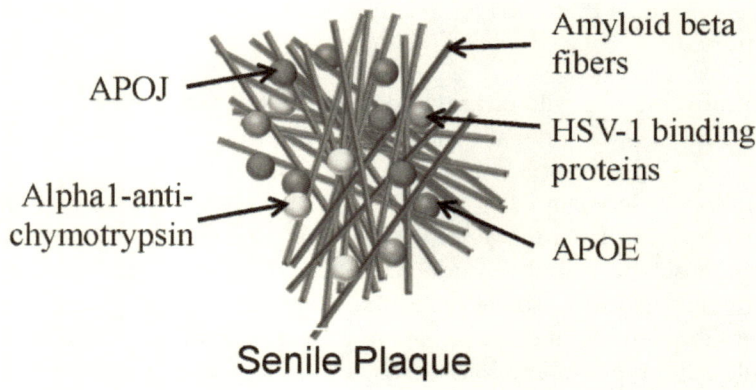

Figure 6.5. The major components of senile plaques.
APOE, apolipoprotein E; APOJ, apolipoprotein J; HSV-1,
herpes simplex virus 1.

As shown in Figure 6.5, some of the proteins that are commonly found in senile plaques include the apolipoproteins E and J which will be covered in more detail later when we discuss genes linked to Alzheimer's disease (Chapters 12 and 13). Other proteins such as alpha1-antichymotrypsin and many herpes simplex virus 1 binding proteins are also present. Alpha1-antichymotrypsin is an inhibitor of an enzyme (chymotrypsin) that digests proteins. It is produced by the pancreas and involved in day-to-day protein digestion in our intestines. But how it functions in amyloid plaques remains a mystery. This is just one more example of a good protein associated with a bad event.

This short protein list is just the tip of this Alzheimer's disease iceberg called the senile plaque. Now let's take a more detailed look at the herpes simplex virus proteins because this virus is well known to many and it is also associated with the disease. But first, for those who would like a refresher course, a short look at the difference between proteins and peptides is covered in the section "FYI: Proteins vs. Peptides".

* * *

FYI: Proteins vs. Peptides

Proteins are made up of long chains of amino acids. Both amyloid beta and tau are each made up of amino acids but this doesn't make them both proteins. Amino acids are joined together by peptide bonds, hence the terms peptide and polypeptide are used when the chain is not big or complex enough to be called a protein. If you think of a protein as a necklace made of pop beads, the amino acids are the beads. The following figure (Figure 6.6) shows a diagram of a small theoretical protein containing all 20 different amino acids (different-colored "beads"). While the pop bead necklace can be folded in many three-dimensional patterns, each normal protein has specific ways it can fold. The way it folds allows it to stay in solution and do its work. If it doesn't fold properly, as discussed earlier in the chapter, it can cause problems. Just as important, the amino acids that are present and their positioning are central to localizing proteins, regulating their activity and affecting to what they can bind.

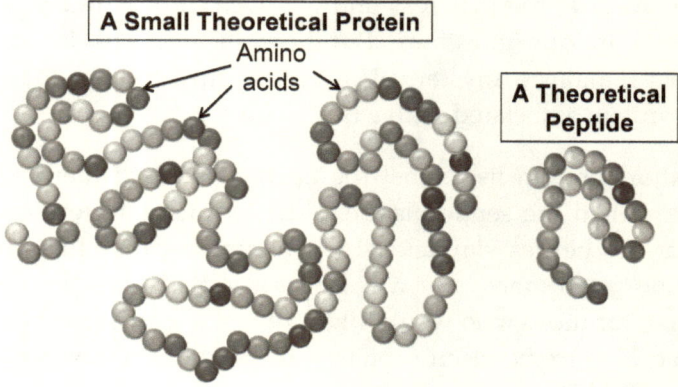

Figure 6.6. A theoretical protein and peptide.

Events that we will mention, like phosphorylation of amino acids within proteins, can change the shape of certain proteins and also alter their function or activity. Phosphorylation is a normal and critical event that is central to the functioning of all cells in our bodies. In fact millions of phosphorylations are occurring in our cells every millisecond of every day. As Martha Stewart might say, "And that's a good thing." As we will see, phosphorylation can be a negative event if it occurs in the wrong protein at the wrong time.

By our pop bead necklace analogy, amyloid beta is a short length of beads. Amyloid beta commonly ranges in size from 39–43 amino acids depending on how it is processed. As we will see, the 42-amino-acid from of amyloid beta (Aβ42) is the most concerning. Because it is a relatively short chain of amino acids, amyloid beta is called a peptide. A short sequence of amino acids is always referred to as a peptide. A theoretical peptide containing 21 amino acids is shown in Figure 6.6. Amyloid beta 42 would be twice this size.

There are many kinds of peptides that work in our bodies, ranging in size from just a few amino acids to a few dozen. They regulate many normal functions throughout our tissues and organs. That said, by peptide standards Aβ42 is a relatively large peptide. Tau, on the other hand, is a full-fledged protein. So a protein is a long chain of amino acids which has folded into a specific shape. Having mentioned phosphorylation, we will see that it plays a central role in the way tau functions.

* * *

Herpes Virus Proteins Are Found in Plaques

There are many lines of evidence that link herpes simplex infections with Alzheimer's disease. In day-to-day life, herpes simplex virus 1 (HSV-1) causes cold sores in humans. With a herpes infection, the virus ultimately enters the brain via nerve cells (typically the trigeminal nerve) where it targets specific brain regions. The virus usually remains dormant in the cell bodies (cytoplasm) of nerve cells until stress or other conditions activate it. This causes virus particles to be made, resulting in a cold sore.

Herpes simplex virus 1 has been shown to induce amyloid beta deposition, the precursor event to amyloid plaque formation. It is also known to cause the phosphorylation of tau protein which leads to neurofibrillary tangle formation, which is detailed in Chapter 7. Similarly, infection with herpes simplex virus 1 can also lead to the loss of neurons from the hippocampus as well as cerebral shrinkage in non-Alzheimer's individuals that is similar to those events in Alzheimer's disease. Finally, herpes simplex virus 1 infections may play a role in Alzheimer's by interacting with other proteins that are linked to the disease, such as apolipoprotein E (APOE). While all of these links are compelling on their own, the true tale comes out when we look at the complement of herpes virus proteins that are present in amyloid plaques.

Dozens of herpes simplex virus 1 proteins that are involved in reproducing more of the viruses have been found in both plaques and tangles. These are primarily binding and processing proteins for virus formation but herpes simplex virus 1 DNA has also been found to occur in plaques as well as in neurofibrillary tangles. One point of view is that these proteins are evidence of the body's fight against herpes simplex virus 1 infections. In fact, it has been said by one group of researchers that the senile plaque is a "cemetery" for the battle between the herpes virus and human cells. Such statements by frontline biomedical researchers only serve to reveal how poor our understanding of Alzheimer's plaques and tangles is and how much more work remains to be done. So let's take a look at the current hypothesis about plaques that dominates the Alzheimer's landscape.

The Amyloid Hypothesis: An In-Depth Look

The formation of amyloid plaques is the first major event that defines Alzheimer's disease. Since these plaques are predominantly fibrous aggregates of fibers of the amyloid beta (Aβ) peptide, this has led to formulation of the "amyloid hypothesis". In other words, the amyloid hypothesis is based upon the presence of protein aggregates called amyloid plaques in the brains of Alzheimer's individuals. Simply stated, the amyloid hypothesis argues that the release of amyloid beta peptides leads to the formation of amyloid beta plaques which in turn lead to the underlying brain changes that characterize Alzheimer's disease. However, the devil is in the details so we need to take a couple of steps back to see exactly how beta amyloid peptides themselves are formed.

* * *

FYI: Amyloid Beta Terminology

Throughout this volume we use the term "amyloid beta" which in research articles is typically written "amyloid β" or "Aβ". The terms "beta-amyloid", "β-amyloid", and "Abeta" are also used to denote this peptide. When we use the term amyloid beta, for the most part we are referring to it in a general sense. However there are two specific forms of amyloid beta that are the most important in Alzheimer's. These are peptides of 40 and 42 amino acids referred to as Aβ40 and Aβ42, respectively, which we will refer to in certain sections of the book. In reviews and research articles these can also be written as $A\beta_{40}$ and $A\beta_{42}$. Alternatively, they can be denoted as $A\beta1_{1-40}$ and $A\beta_{1-42}$. In older papers, "beta amyloid" was frequently used but now its use is less common. These alternative forms are used for different reasons. Some are just conventions of the journal in which the papers are published while others are used to be more precise reflections of the peptides in question.

* * *

If senile plaques are made from amyloid beta peptides, those peptides have to come from somewhere. The whole process begins with a protein that is lodged in nerve cell membranes. It is called amyloid precursor protein, or APP, for short. Amyloid precursor protein is a membrane-bound protein that gets cut up successively by two enzymes with the resulting release of one small amyloid beta peptide. The basic events in processing of amyloid precursor protein to release amyloid beta are shown in Figure 6.7. At first an enzyme called beta-secretase (BACE1) cuts the protein, releasing most of it from the cell membrane. This leaves a short chunk of the protein still stuck in the membrane. At this point the second enzyme, gamma-secretase, cuts the remaining piece causing the release of the amyloid beta fragment to the outside of the cell, plus the release of another small piece inside the cell. We are only interested in the small amyloid beta peptide because, as duly noted, this is the nasty little peptide that is the basic component of plaque formation in Alzheimer's disease. For those who are interested, these events are explained in much more detail in the supplementary section "FYI: The Pathways Leading to Amyloid Beta".

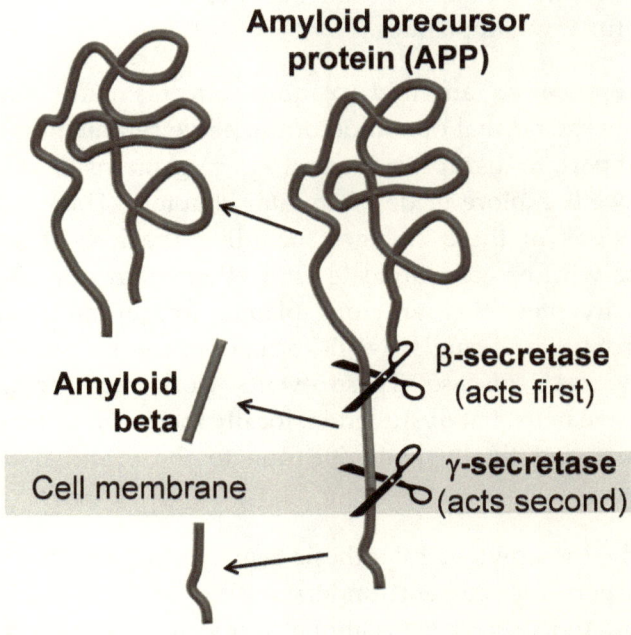

Figure 6.7. Two enzymes (beta-secretase and gamma-secretase) work in sequence to release amyloid beta peptides from amyloid precursor protein.

In reality, due to a number of genetic factors and processing events, more than one form of amyloid beta can be produced. These peptides can range in size from 17–46 amino acids in length. However, as detailed above (FYI: Amyloid Beta Terminology) the amyloidogenic pathway that leads to plaque formation predominantly produces amyloid beta peptides of 40 amino acids or 42 amino acids in length (i.e., Aβ40 and Aβ42, respectively). While the 40-amino-acid form is the most predominant (90% of peptide produced), the accumulated evidence argues that the 42-amino-acid amyloid beta (Aβ42) is the more toxic fragment of the two species with respect to Alzheimer's pathology.

Thus the amyloid hypothesis suggests that the increased production of amyloid beta is the initiator of the pathological cascade that leads to Alzheimer's disease. This cascade begins with production and then the spontaneous aggregation of amyloid peptides that, as detailed above, results in the formation of harmful amyloid plaques.

The presence of amyloid plaques affects many functions, especially the normal operation of the nerve cell membrane. This leads, in part, to disruptive increases in calcium inside the cells, a subject we'll explore in detail in later chapters. There are many ramifications of these changes including the loss of ability to associate with or communicate with other brain cells. It is now widely accepted that amyloid plaque formation is followed by neurofibrillary tangle (NFT) formation, the second hallmark of Alzheimer's disease. These events work together to cause progressive neuronal dysfunction, locally increased inflammatory responses, and finally dementia due to the eventual death of neurons.

Arguably, the amyloid hypothesis remains the dominant theory based upon the current understanding of how Alzheimer's develops, and so most translational research has been focused on the development of therapeutic strategies aimed at reducing the amount of amyloid beta (especially Aβ42) that is formed. However, by the time plaques, tangles and the neurological symptoms appear, it is too late to reverse the amount of neuronal loss or to halt the disease.

* * *

FYI: The Pathways Leading to Amyloid Beta

The route leading to amyloid beta formation is called the amyloidogenic (amyloid-forming) pathway. It is very well defined so let's take a deeper look at it (Figure 6.8).

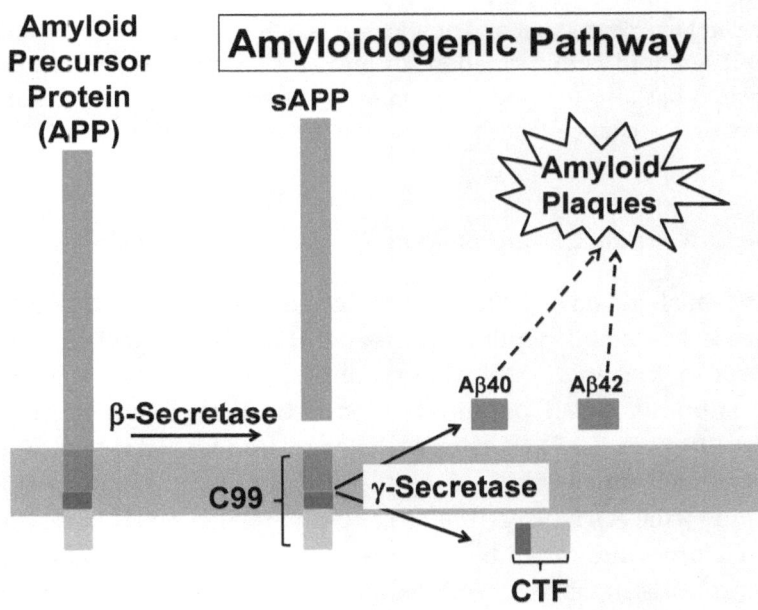

Figure 6.8. The proteolytic processing of amyloid beta precursor protein (APP).

Amyloid beta production in neurons requires an initial cleavage of amyloid precursor protein (APP) by the enzyme beta-secretase. This enzyme action releases a large extracellular soluble APP (sAPP) fragment, leaving behind a shorter membrane-bound fragment (C99) that is ~99 amino acids in length. The C99 transmembrane fragment is then cleaved by the enzyme gamma-secretase to produce either of two major amyloid beta fragments: $A\beta40$ or $A\beta42$ (other $A\beta$ species have also been identified). At the same time, a non-harmful C-terminal fragment (CTF) is released inside of the cell. Gamma-secretase is composed of four proteins: nicastrin, presenilin-1/-2, presenilin enhancer protein-2 (PEN-2) and the anterior pharynx defective-1 (Aph-1) protein (discussed in Chapter 12).

There is also a more common pathway that has nothing to do with causing Alzheimer's disease. It is the non-amyloidogenic pathway in which APP is cut by alpha-secretase, not beta-secretase. This pathway is essential for the normal functioning of cells. In this process, the enzyme alpha-secretase cleaves inside of the amyloid beta region, precluding the formation of the harmful amyloid beta peptides. The resulting membrane-bound sequence is then cleaved by gamma-secretase to release non-amyloidogenic peptides. In spite of the excellent current state of knowledge, much remains to be learned about amyloid beta formation. In terms of controlling Alzheimer's, research has also focused on enhancing the role of alpha-secretase to decrease the chance that the amyloid beta peptides can form.

* * *

The End-Product Troublemaker

So when all is said and done, the molecule of interest in Alzheimer's disease is a small peptide consisting of 42 amino acids. So let's take a look at this nasty little piece of protein. Amino acids are the subunits of all proteins and can be designated by single letters (e.g., A, L, F) or as three-letter codes (e.g., Ala, Leu, Phe). These short forms stand for the full name of the amino acid: alanine (Ala, A), leucine (L, Leu) and phenylalanine (F, Phe). Both short forms are used by scientists to denote the 20 common amino acids in cells. If we look at the following figure, both the single- and three-letter codes for all of the 42 amino acids of amyloid beta 42 are shown (Figure 6.9). Between them is a three-dimensional model showing the shape of the protein.

Of course, as the old joke goes, there won't be a test later on this. However, it is interesting to put a face, albeit a dastardly one, to one of the key molecules linked to the onset and progression of Alzheimer's disease. One of the perplexing issues is why this specific sequence is so harmful. What makes it organize into the disruptive and harmful amyloid plaques that appear in the Alzheimer's brain?

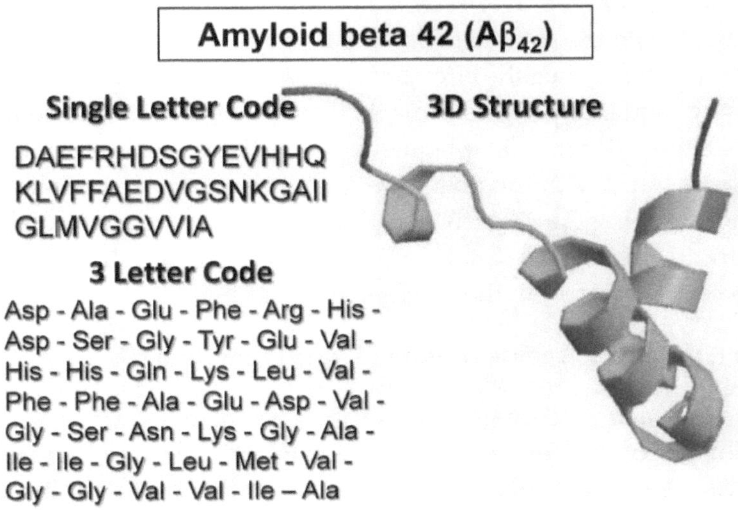

Figure 6.9. The 3D structure and amino acid composition of amyloid beta 42.

A Controversial Current View

While there is no doubt that the presence of amyloid plaques in the brain has devastating effects, there is some doubt about their importance as the true causative agents of Alzheimer's disease. This is an emerging story that we'll comment on here but which will undoubtedly continue to be unraveled as biomedical research continues. First of all, the appearance of amyloid beta and its transition into amyloid plaques is not an early event or the cause of Alzheimer's disease—many believe it occurs after the onset of the disease has already been set in motion. It is also considered by many researchers that the initial formation of amyloid beta is a defense mechanism by brain cells. In other words, the production of the peptide is meant to help cells rather than hurt them.

So workers are focusing on what might occur before the amyloid peptides appear. An early event in the onset of Alzheimer's disease is oxidative stress. Oxidative stress is caused by the release of reactive oxygen species within cells, as detailed in Chapter 15 of this book. Amyloid beta 42, which has antioxidant attributes, may be over-secreted initially to counteract oxidative stress. While the soluble form may be initially protective of nerve cells and counteract the effects of oxidative stress, their subsequent aggregation into plaques turns them toxic. Regardless, as detailed in Chapter 8, amyloid plaques will continue to be a target for drug therapy with the goal of reducing plaque load and slowing if not stopping the cognitive decline linked to Alzheimer's disease. With this in mind, let's take a preliminary look at what might be the very first event in the disease.

Do Nucleating Agents Initiate Plaque Formation?

As has been said many times, amyloid plaques are a central hallmark of Alzheimer's disease. Amyloid peptides undergo a series of changes ultimately forming fibrils that organize into plaques containing a diversity of other proteins and cellular molecules. The question that remains to be answered is, "How does this all start?" To date it is not known how the first amyloid peptides begin their wayward journey towards plaque formation. It is known that they accumulate and grow. It is not known why they accumulate in specific areas or how they begin to cluster in these regions.

One topic that is often not discussed is the potential role for a nucleating agent that starts amyloid plaque formation. Nucleating agents are substances that initiate specific events. We've all heard about "seeding" clouds to cause rain to fall. When you open a bottle of pop, this initiates the formation of bubbles of carbon dioxide. Stick your finger in a glass of soda pop and the nucleation of CO_2 bubbles will occur on your fingers. Of course, this event can be made more dramatic as shown in the numerous YouTube™ videos of what happens when a Mentos™ candy is dropped into a bottle of Coca Cola™. Crystals form by nucleation as well. In the cell there are many well-known examples of nucleation, especially in the way the cell's cytoskeleton (e.g., actin, microtubules) forms. So it is possible that some as-yet-undiscovered cellular molecule starts the condensation of amyloid peptides into amyloid plaques.

Chapter 7

The Tangled Web

A Scientific Battle

In the previous chapter, the importance of amyloid beta plaques as a primary indicator of Alzheimer's disease was detailed. Here we will look at the second defining attribute of Alzheimer's disease: tangles. While amyloid plaques form outside of Alzheimer's brain cells, neurofibrillary tangles form inside of them. A decade or so ago the relationship between amyloid beta and tau, the major constituent of neurofibrillary tangles, and the importance of each one was not well understood. At that time a battle was raging between the two conflicting theories of Alzheimer's disease.

This academic war was between those who believed tau was the primary agent causing Alzheimer's disease and those who favored beta amyloid as the initiating culprit. While we use the term amyloid beta, this peptide is also referred as beta amyloid (βA) leading one scientific comedian to refer to this non-religious disagreement as the "Tauists vs. the Baptists". In the end the beta amyloid group or "Baptists" won out. It is now widely held that the formation of amyloid plaques precedes the appearance of neurofibrillary tangles in Alzheimer's brain cells. While tau has been shown to be a later event in the progression of Alzheimer's, it is no less important than amyloid beta in defining the disease.

Tau and Neurodegeneration

Neurofibrillary tangles are not just a defining attribute of Alzheimer's disease but are found in other neurodegenerative diseases as well. It has been well documented that the protein responsible for these tangles underlies a number of neurodegenerative events. The protein is called "tau" like the 19th letter of the Greek alphabet. For a medium-sized protein, tau packs quite a punch in normal cells as well as in a number of different neurodegenerative diseases. Because of the presence of tau inclusions, these neurodegenerative diseases are collectively known as taupathies (also commonly called tauopathies). They include the well-known Pick's disease, some forms of Parkinson's disease and Alzheimer's disease. Other less well-known disorders such as certain prion diseases and chronic traumatic encephalopathy are also classed as taupathies.

In Alzheimer's, the tau protein is phosphorylated. Phosphate groups are added to certain amino acids in the protein. In fact, so many amino acids get phosphate groups attached that tau is said to be hyperphosphorylated. When this occurs it causes tau to organize into neurofibrillary tangles (NFTs) inside of nerve cells. Before we get into how these tangles arise and how they are linked to Alzheimer's disease, we will look at what tau normally does in cells because this should yield insight into what happens when tau is altered.

Tangles in the Brain

As their name implies, neurofibrillary tangles are like knots in one's hair—they are fibrous tangles of protein. The question now is, "What exactly is tau protein and how does it make tangles in the brain?" In normal cells tau is involved in organizing part of the cytoskeleton of our cells. It binds specifically to components called microtubules. "What the heck are microtubules?" you now might ask. To answer this question, we need to review some of the biology we learned in school. So here's a short discourse on microtubules.

As their name implies, microtubules look like small ("micro") pipes or tubes ("tubule"). Microtubules form part of every cell's internal skeleton, more commonly referred to as its cytoskeleton. The word is derived from "cyto" (as in cytoplasm) and, of course, "skeleton". As such, like our skeleton, microtubules are involved in maintaining the shape of the cell and how it moves (Figure 7.1). As we all learned in biology class, they are also part of the spindle apparatus that moves chromosomes during cell division. In humans, microtubules also form the central part of cilia in the lungs and female genital tract and the flagellum of sperm cells.

Microtubule Patterns in Different Cell Types

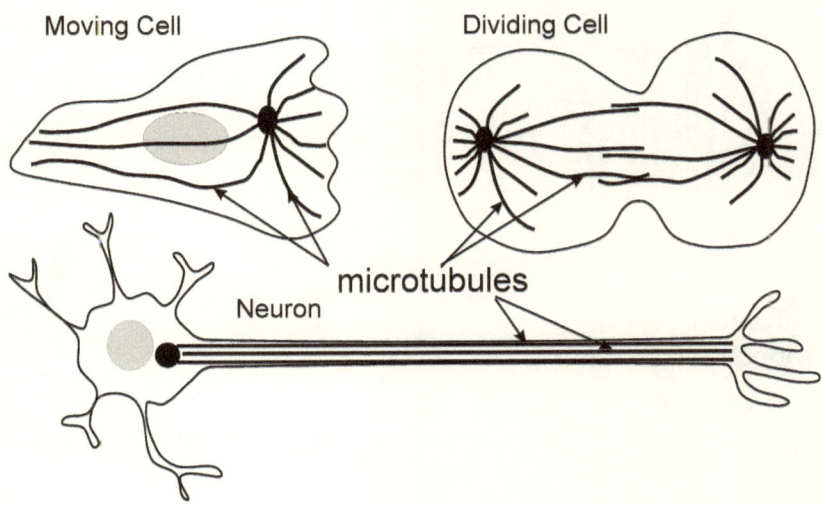

Figure 7.1. The pattern of microtubules in different cell types.

Of interest to us as we continue to delve into the causes of Alzheimer's, microtubules maintain the elongated axons that allow nerve cells to extend over long distances to regulate muscle contractions, interactions with other nerves and more. As we will see, microtubules have even more functions—and those appear to be central to the role of tau in neurodegeneration. For example, microtubules direct neurosecretion, the release of neurotransmitters as mentioned in Chapter 5, which allows nerve cells in the brain to communicate with other brain cells. To get to the role of tau, we need to look even closer at microtubules.

Tau Binds to Microtubules

When we examine microtubules using the electron microscope, they look like long, relatively straight rubber hoses (Figure 7.2). If you cut across them, just like a hose they have a wall and a central space called a lumen (a common term also used for spaces in cells, tissues and organs). Unlike a hose, there is no proof anything runs through the lumen—all the functions occur at the surface of microtubules. One of the proteins on the surface of microtubules is tau.

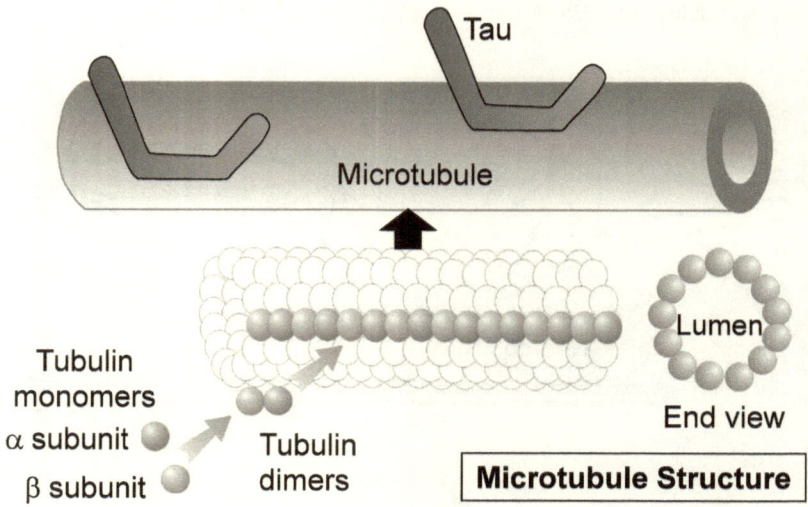

Figure 7.2. The structure of microtubules.
(From O'Day, 2012. *Introduction to the Human Cell —
The Unit of Life and Disease*, an eBook)

As shown in the figures above and below, tau binds to microtubules (Figures 7.2, 7.3). Tau, in fact, was first identified as a microtubule assembly factor. The wall of the microtubule is made up of tubulin subunits, so to make one is like putting together a set of Lego™ blocks where tau serves as the platform on which to start the building process. It may also cross-link microtubules as shown in Figure 7.3. While tau also serves other functions, it clearly has an effect on the formation and organization of microtubules which in turn has impact on how nerve cells function. Tau does this by binding to microtubules via special microtubule-binding domains (MBDs) that are present within the tau protein. These binding domains are specific sequences of amino acids in the protein. While biochemists know the amino acid sequences of the microtubule-binding domains for the various forms of tau that exist, all these details won't help us understand the basis of how tau is linked to neurodegeneration. For that we do need to understand how good tau can be turned bad.

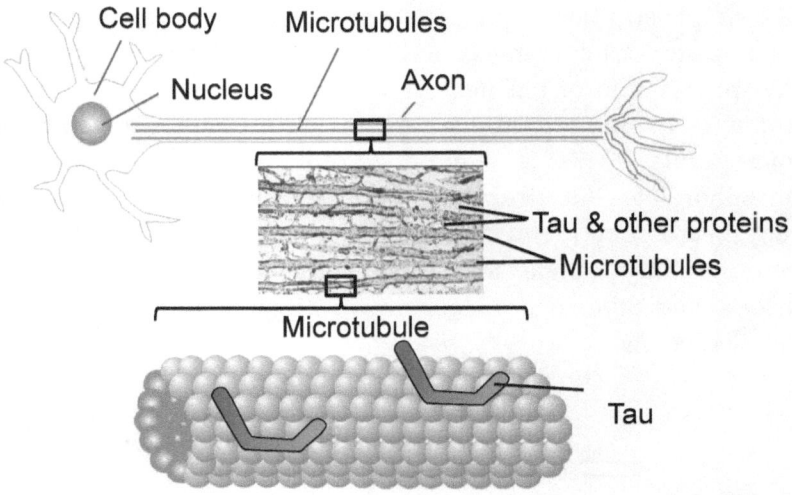

Figure 7.3. The organization of microtubules and tau in neurons. (From O'Day, 2012. *Introduction to the Human Cell — The Unit of Life and Disease*, an eBook)

Good Tau Can Be Turned Bad

Most proteins can be altered once they are made. This can be done in a number of ways. Because tau can be altered in so many different ways, we'll list some of these before we focus on the most studied alteration that is believed to be central to Alzheimer's disease. Tau can undergo phosphorylation (phosphate groups added in specific places), acetylation (acetyl groups added), glycosylation (sugar groups added), ubiquitylation (ubiquitin added) and sumoylation (sumo proteins are added). Since these aren't all of the changes that can be made, you get some idea of the complexity of events that are related to tau. These alterations happen to many other proteins as well and this is just one of the reasons trying to understand changes in cells that happen during any disease is tremendously difficult. The good news is that this complexity also reveals potential targets for developing new Alzheimer's therapies. Having said that, let's look at the primary culprit in making tau a bad protein. That culprit is phosphorylation. While we summarize events here, a more detailed explanation of protein phosphorylation is covered below (FYI: Phosphorylation: A Critical Life Process).

The simple addition of phosphate groups to tau proteins changes them from cellular angels into devilish Alzheimer's proteins. Phosphorylation of tau near or within the microtubule-binding domain, mentioned above, makes tau unable to bind to microtubules. This is summarized in Figure 7.4. Once the phosphorylated tau (P-tau) is removed from the microtubules it can then begin the complex sequence of events leading to neurofibrillary tangle formation, a hallmark of Alzheimer's disease and other neurodegenerative diseases. These events are detailed below.

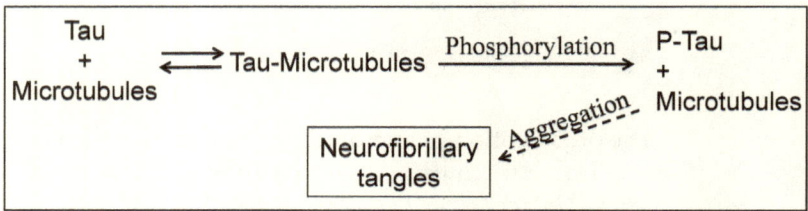

Figure 7.4. The link between tau, microtubules and neurofibrillary tangle formation.

Tau in Neurons

So if phosphorylated tau leads to neurofibrillary tangles which in turn are related to neurodegeneration, we need to delve further into its specific function in neurons. Neurons have a cell body from which one or more axons extend. (For simplicity, throughout this book we've been looking primarily at a brain neuron that has only one long axon.) Essentially all of the critical molecules for the survival and function of all nerve cells are made in the cell body. To get to the synapse where stimulation of other nerves will occur, these molecules must travel the long distance from the cell body along the axon to the nerve endings. As shown in the following figure, tau is specifically localized within the axon while another microtubule-associated protein (MAP-2) localizes to the cell body (Figure 7.5; Note also this nerve cell has three axons).

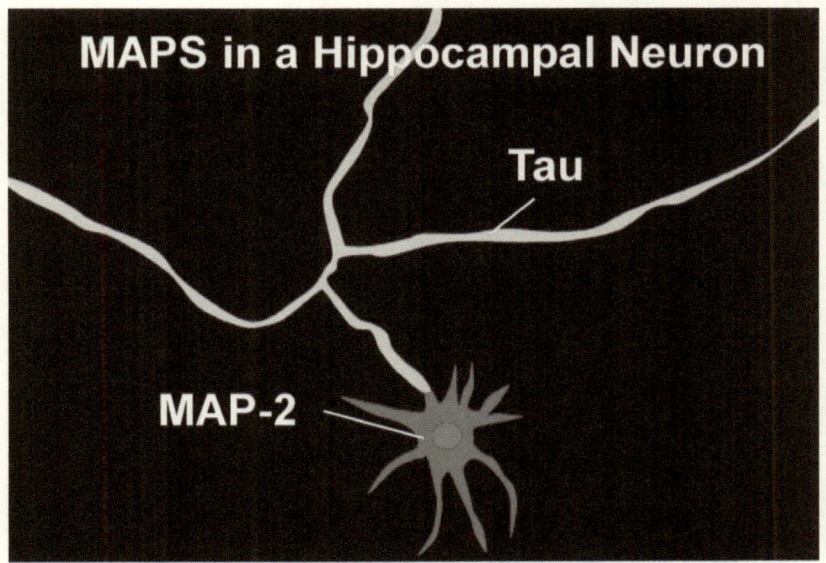

Figure 7.5. Tau localizes to axons while another microtubule-associated protein (MAP-2) is localized in the cell body of neurons. (From O'Day, 2012. *Introduction to the Human Cell—The Unit of Life and Disease*, an eBook)

In spite of the distances that have to be covered, the events in nerve cells occur within milliseconds. Clearly diffusion would not be an efficient way to move molecules and other cellular components quickly from one end of a neuron to the other. To deal with this, the cell has evolved a railroad-type system wherein molecules are transported along the protein railway tracks both to and from the synapse. The railroad tracks along which molecules are transported are made up of microtubules as indicated in the following picture (Figure 7.6) and as detailed above.

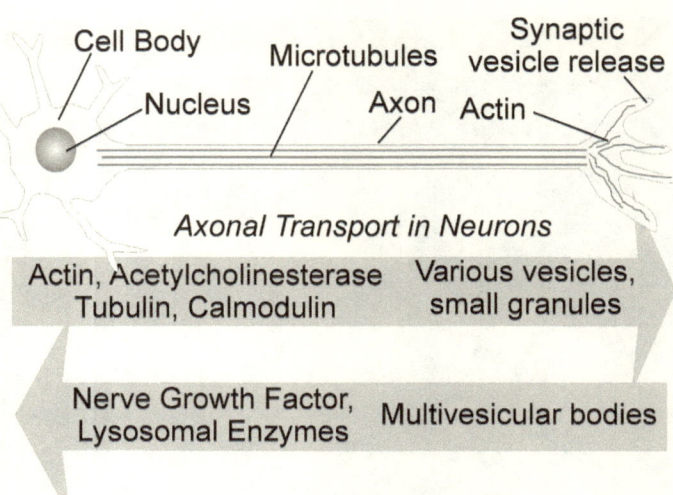

Figure 7.6. Molecules and other cellular components move to and from the cell body along microtubules in nerve axons. (Modified from O'Day, 2012. *Introduction to the Human Cell — The Unit of Life and Disease*, an eBook)

The directional movement of some of the molecules is also shown in the large arrows in Figure 7.6 that appear below the picture of the neuron. For example, certain molecules (e.g., actin, tubulin) and cellular constituents (e.g., vesicles, granules) are primarily moved from the cell body to the synapse. Others (e.g., nerve growth factor, lysosomal enzymes, and multivesicular bodies) are transported in the opposite direction. So microtubules not only maintain the elongated shape of the axon, they also provide a transport system (like railway tracks) for moving molecules as well as various other cellular constituents to and from the synapse. These events are central to nerve cell function.

Because tau is localized in the axons and because transport along microtubules in these axons is central to nerve function, clearly removing tau and disrupting microtubule function would affect nerve cell function. In the Alzheimer's brain, the phosphorylation of tau causes it to be released from microtubules. It can now start to form neurofibrillary tangles. In addition, the loss of tau can disrupt the microtubule functions discussed above leading to faulty nerve cell function. Thus the phosphorylation of tau has more than one effect in Alzheimer's disease. As a result, tau phosphorylation is the target for research aimed at developing effective pharmaceuticals to combat Alzheimer's disease.

* * *

FYI: Phosphorylation: A Critical Life Process

As we work through this chapter, we will see that, like the processing and deposition of amyloid, the process of tau phosphorylation and neurofibrillary tangle formation is complex and just as significant. Scientists have identified some of the enzymes that are responsible, but not all of them. We'll first look at the general processes of adding phosphate groups to proteins and removing them. Then we will see which specific enzymes do these things in brain cells.

As mentioned above, the process of addition and removal of phosphate groups is a continual ongoing event in all of our cells, tissues and organs. Without phosphorylation, we would die. This seems a bit contradictory because phosphorylation of the wrong proteins, such as tau, can also kill us.

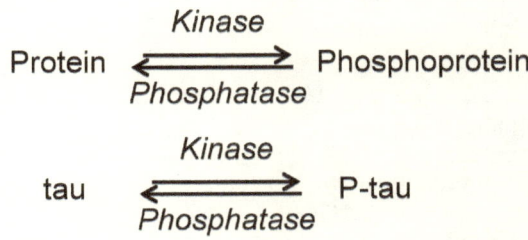

Figure 7.7. Kinases add phosphate groups to proteins while phosphatases remove them.

Enzymes that add phosphate groups to other proteins, turning them into phosphoproteins, are generally referred to as kinases (Figure 7.7). This is apparently derived from the word "<u>kin</u>etic" which denotes energetic movement or activity, and the suffix "-ase" which typically indicates an enzyme. As we will see there are many kinases that can add phosphate groups to tau, transforming it into P-tau (phosphorylated tau). There are fewer enzymes that are known to remove phosphate groups from this protein. The enzymes that take phosphate groups off proteins and other molecules are typically referred to as phosphatases (i.e., phosphate-removing enzymes [-ases]) (Figure 7.7). Thus the amount of tau and P-tau is dependent on the amounts of phosphorylation and dephosphorylation that are occurring at any time. Based on the level of phosphorylation, tau can then go through a progressive accumulation that ultimately can lead to neurofibrillary tangle formation.

* * *

Tau Phosphorylation Gets Hyper!

The formation of neurofibrillary tangles begins with the phosphorylation of tau and progresses through a well-defined sequence of events. As shown in Figure 7.8, the phosphorylation of tau by kinases leads to P-tau which can then organize as dimers (pairs of proteins). At this stage, dephosphorylation by phosphatases, as discussed below and above (FYI: Phosphorylation: A Critical Life Process), can prevent dimer formation by converting tau back to its unphosphorylated status. However with the continued phosphorylation of tau, the P-tau dimers aggregate together in groups of many phosphorylated tau proteins. This is the hyperphosphorylation state of tau. The hyperphosphorylated tau proteins in turn can now organize into filaments.

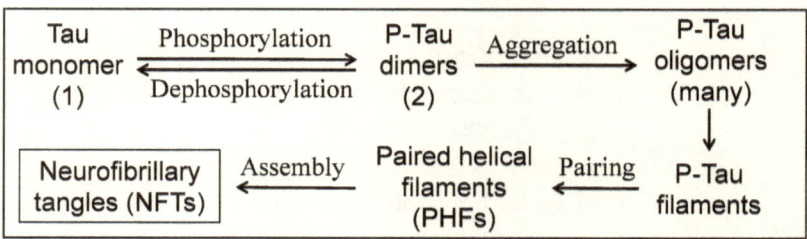

Figure 7.8. The sequence of events in the formation of neurofibrillary tangles.

This stage is followed by pairing of the filaments which, in keeping with their formation, are called paired helical filaments (PHFs). These in turn assemble into the final neurofibrillary tangles. During assembly other proteins are added as well, making the final neurofibrillary tangles a mixture of hyperphosphorylated tau filaments and other constituents.

Tau Phosphorylation: Identifying the Culprits

As one might expect, scientists have been working out the details of this sequence of events for decades. They are trying to find out which kinases and phosphatases are important because they could serve as pharmaceutical targets. Scientists are also trying to understand how these different stages occur because therapies could be developed and used to stop the process in its tracks at whatever stage the disease has reached. Clearly the most appealing target is the initial pairing to form dimers and the aggregation of these dimers to form oligomers but that means early detection is required. By preventing the initiation of tangle formation, it might be possible to prevent some of the early events of neurodegeneration. Of course there's also hope that interfering with the later stages could also be helpful in halting the progression of aspects associated with the late stages of Alzheimer's disease. Thus preventing filament formation, their pairing to form paired helical filaments and their final assembly into neurofibrillary tangles each hold out hope for therapeutic development. The section "FYI: Untangling Tau with Just a Few Phosphatases" describes the action of kinases and phosphatases on tau in more detail. Then we'll look a bit more at the neurofibrillary tangles assembly process as a target of research.

* * *

FYI: Untangling Tau with Just a Few Phosphatases

Tau from Alzheimer's brains has been shown to be phosphorylated at over two dozen different places. So, as mentioned above, it's not just phosphorylated—it is hyperphosphorylated. In reality there are over six dozen potential phosphorylation sites, some of which are phosphorylated in tau from normal brains, some from Alzheimer's brains and some from both. Some amino acids haven't yet been proven to be phosphorylated at any time. Although there are 20 different amino acids that are commonly found in proteins, tau is phosphorylated on only two different amino acids that are localized in many places within the protein. These amino acids are serine and threonine. Thankfully, the general term for the enzymes that phosphorylate these two amino acid targets is "serine/threonine kinases". Similarly, the enzymes that remove the phosphate groups from these amino acids are called "serine/threonine phosphatases".

Sometimes scientists actually pick terms that make sense! Updating Figure 7.7, the events of tau phosphorylation and dephosphorylation are shown in Figure 7.9. So let's start with the phosphatases that dephosphorylate tau because they comprise a much smaller group.

Actually, we are talking about a very small group of one or two which I realize is too small to be a group. Of these enzymes, serine/threonine phosphatase-2A (PP-2A) has been identified as the most active one that dephosphorylates tau in the brain, potentially transforming it from abnormal, phosphorylated tau to normal tau. In the Alzheimer's brain, PP-2A enzyme activity is decreased so it is less effective at removing phosphate groups from tau. If PP-2A activity is inhibited in normal brain cells in mice by the addition of pharmacological agents, then hyperphosphorylation of tau occurs. Thus PP-2A has been proven to be directly linked to the phosphorylation status of tau in the brain.

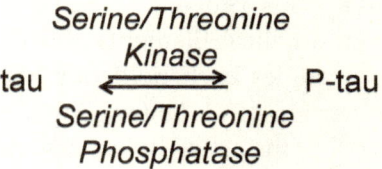

Figure 7.9. Serine/threonine kinases phosphorylate tau while serine/threonine phosphatases dephosphorylate P-tau.

A second tau phosphatase has also been identified. It is also a serine/threonine phosphatase but it is different because it is regulated by calcium. (We'll talk about the central role of calcium when we discuss "The Calcium Hypothesis" of Alzheimer's disease in Chapter 16.) This second enzyme is serine/threonine phosphatase-2B (PP-2B). It was originally called calcineurin because its activity is regulated by calcium (hence "calci") and it was discovered in brain tissue (hence "neurin"). PP-2B does many other things in brain cells and is linked to Alzheimer's disease in other ways as well. It is also tied to brain development in Down syndrome. We'll come back to this enzyme as well as the incidence of Alzheimer's in Down syndrome individuals in Chapter 12. It's also possible that other phosphatases are involved in Alzheimer's but none have proven to be as central in Alzheimer's disease as PP-2A and, possibly, PP-2B.

* * *

Tangling Tau: A Complex Web of Kinases

The kinase story is much more complex but we can simplify it because, while there are many kinases, they are all serine/threonine kinases. So they can add phosphate groups to serine and/or threonine amino acids in tau. Each of these kinases differs in the amounts that are present in brain cells and how they are regulated, among other things. So after we list the usual suspects, we'll focus on just a few of the major players in the neurofibrillary tangle story. This is because when you distill it all down, the role of these various kinases in neurofibrillary tangle formation and the way research work is being done to prevent their function is fundamentally the same.

Although many kinases are suspected to play a role in Alzheimer's disease, only four of them appear to be of prime importance and thus have been well studied. These enzymes and the results of their phosphorylation of tau are shown in Figure 7.10. Their names are glycogen synthase kinase 3 beta (GSK-3β), cyclin-dependent kinase 5 (CDK5), mitogen-activated protein kinase (MAPK), and microtubule affinity-regulating kinase (MARK).

These names do not evoke a feeling that the enzymes are strictly related to Alzheimer's disease. This is because most proteins and enzymes in the cell serve many functions. Thus, glycogen synthase kinase is involved in regulating sugar levels in the body. Since that was its first discovered function, that's why it was named is this way. The same is true for the other enzymes which were named for the functions they initially were found to carry out or regulate.

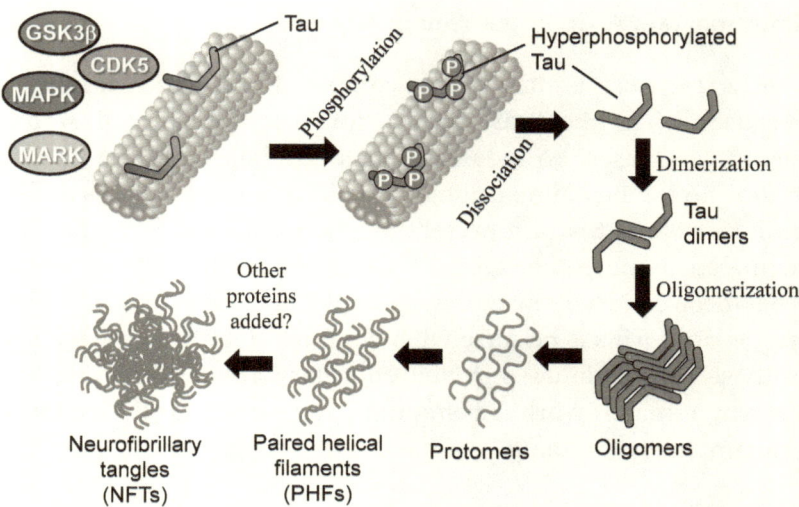

Figure 7.10. Serine/threonine kinases phosphorylate tau while serine/threonine phosphatases dephosphorylate P-tau.

The action of these enzymes leads to the hyperphosphorylation of tau which causes it to be released from microtubules. The hyperphosphorylated tau then goes through a series of changes as introduced above (Figure 7.8) but elaborated upon further in Figure 7.10. Thus freed from microtubules, tau dimers form which are transformed to oligomers. The oligomers line up to form protomers which pair up as the paired helical filaments introduced above. These filaments then organize along with other proteins and cellular components to form neurofibrillary tangles—the tangles that are characteristic of the Alzheimer's brain.

Clearly, it is not important for the reader to memorize all of these different enzymes and the events that lead to tangle formation. But it is important to be aware of the complexity of what is being studied and the proteins that are involved in forming the tangles linked to Alzheimer's disease. In the long run it will enhance our grasp of just how difficult it is to find cures for a debilitating disease of any type.

Tau and the Mind of a Mouse

Much of tau's responsibilities in the cell were revealed by scientists who took cells apart using a diversity of methods. This allowed them to learn where tau protein localizes and what it does. This in turn led to all the work on tau and its association with microtubules as summarized above. Other work revealed that tau does many other things and binds to other cellular components as well. Much of this work was generated through the use of knockout mutants in mouse. The use of gene knockouts has provided major insights into what proteins do in normal and diseased cells. Without getting too academic, it's important to understand what a knockout mutant is. We all know that genes code for proteins. During embryonic development and throughout our lives, genes are turned on and off to make the proteins our cells need to change and to function.

We've learned through history that some people are missing certain functional genes. For example, Tay-Sachs disease is due to the loss of function of a single protein because of a genetic mutation. This leads to neurological and other problems and early death. All because of a single mutant gene! In fact we are all mutants. All of our genes are full of mutations but most of them are irrelevant because they don't functionally change the proteins they encode. Once in a while, a mutation occurs that either stops a gene from producing a required protein or it makes an abnormal protein that doesn't work properly. An example of this is hemophilia. There are two main types of this blood-clotting disorder and they are both caused by mutations in different genes. These mutations result in abnormal factors that are less efficient at causing blood clotting.

Scientists now are able to do the same thing that evolution has done—not with humans but with "model" organisms. One of these model organisms is the mouse. The mouse has long served as a model for understanding a wide diversity of human diseases as well as the specific function of a multitude of proteins. With the development of gene knockouts in mice, their biomedical value increased even more. So what is a gene knockout? As its name implies, a specific gene is knocked out. Like a boxer who is knocked out, the gene can no longer function. Unlike the boxer, however, the gene can never function because it has either been deleted or so damaged that recovering it is impossible.

Scientists use molecular techniques to destroy a specific gene so it cannot make the protein it normally encodes. So the knockout mouse is just like its cloned brothers and sisters except it is missing a single protein. By following the development of the mouse at all levels—tissues, organs and cells—it is possible to find out the importance of that protein. Thus, knockout of tau in mice has led to some new revelations on tau function that may be related to its underlying role in taupathies, including Alzheimer's disease.

While tau was originally considered to be just a microtubule-binding protein, it has now been shown to associate with a number of other components in the cell. It binds to actin filaments, another major cytoskeletal element, to various lipids and to various proteins involved in cell communication. Of particular interest is its association with apolipoprotein E3 or APOE3, a protein that is intimately linked to Alzheimer's disease. The apolipoprotein E is a small protein that is involved in moving cholesterol throughout the body. There are three common forms of the protein: APOE2, APOE3 and APOE4. Mutations in APOE3 have been shown to be involved in some cases of Alzheimer's disease so we'll come back to this protein and its gene later in Chapters 12 and 13.

While the significance of all of these previously unknown associations of tau remains to be elucidated, there is one perplexing result from tau knockouts—no brain defects were detected in embryonic or adult mice. Not only did tau knockout mice have normal-appearing brains, but also they lacked behavioral defects and deficient memory. Thus the loss of tau function is not the actual cause of neuronal dysfunction or neurodegeneration. While that might seem to be a negative result, it can also be interpreted as supporting the role for hyperphosphorylated tau as the culprit in various taupathies such as Alzheimer's disease. In other words, the loss of tau isn't the issue—the appearance of large amounts of altered hyperphosphorylated tau is the problem.

Since knockouts of tau don't cause defects and, in fact, may actually prevent the development of taupathies, researchers are taking the knockout models even further. They are doing this by knocking out not one gene but two and even more genes at the same time, to show which proteins work together with tau to cause taupathies. Scientists have also shown that normal levels of tau as well as of amyloid beta and APOE4 are essential for the development of neuronal and behavioral defects. The question that remains is whether amyloid beta, tau and APOE4 are working together or independently to cause the neurodegenerative events underlying Alzheimer's disease.

Tau Can Move from Neuron to Neuron

As we have seen, Alzheimer's disease spreads through the brain in a specific pattern to sequentially shut down normal neuronal functions (Chapter 4). Exactly how this occurs remained in question until a very recent discovery. Working with mice, researchers showed that tau from one brain neuron could move into nerves in adjacent brain regions. This spread could be the mechanism whereby Alzheimer's disease taupathy moves from one brain region to the next. If this is the way neurodegeneration is propagated, then understanding the exact mechanism by which tau is transferred from cell to cell could provide a target for developing new strategies for stopping the progression of neurodegeneration. That said, scientists still don't understand how this occurs. But that doesn't mean that the answer will be a long time coming—there could be a solution very soon.

So how could such protein transfer occur? All cells can secrete large proteins. Salivary glands secrete proteins as saliva; milk glands in the breast secrete milk proteins. Protein secretion is a normal event, so the secretion of tau could also be a normal cellular process. Since there are existing drugs that affect protein secretion then these drugs might be useful in preventing the spread of tau in the Alzheimer's sufferer if secretion of tau is the problem.

All cells can also take up proteins and other molecules from their outside environment. That's how cholesterol gets into cells. They can do this by taking up extracellular fluid in bulk or by selectively taking up single proteins. There are also pharmaceuticals that can stop these kinds of cell uptake (or endocytosis). Assuming that tau is spread by one neuron taking up tau secreted from another neuron, then maybe these drugs would be of use. However, if the spread of tau is due to cell death, which becomes comparatively rampant in the Alzheimer's brain, then the key is to prevent cell death (apoptosis) which is discussed at the end of Chapter 5. The good news is that having identified how tau moves in the brain has opened the door for potential new therapies. And that's always a good thing.

Chapter 8

Plaques and Tangles as Pharmaceutical Targets

The Major Hypotheses for Alzheimer's Disease

By the summer of 2012, it was reported that over 330 ongoing Alzheimer's disease clinical trials were underway worldwide. This therapeutic landscape for treating Alzheimer's disease has changed significantly over the years. As the search for a cure continues, it has been argued that even slowing the disease has merit. For example, if the onset of the disease could be slowed by a single year, hundreds of thousands fewer cases would develop each year. Thus the development of therapeutic interventions is important not only to the individual but to society as a whole. To understand where clinical research on Alzheimer's disease has been and where it is going, it is important to examine the major hypotheses that dominate the field. In some cases the term "hypothesis" is a bit strong but, in keeping with published work, we'll use this term. These "hypotheses" are summarized in Table 8.1.

A Summary of the Major Hypotheses for Alzheimer's Disease

The Amyloid Hypothesis: The production of amyloid beta and its contribution to amyloid plaque formation leads to the neurodegenerative events of the disease.

The Tau Hypothesis: The phosphorylation of tau protein causes it to form neurofibrillary tangles that cause neurodegeneration in AD.

The Cholinergic Hypothesis: Deficiencies in the neurotransmitter acetylcholine underlie the causes and symptoms of AD.

The Calcium Hypothesis: The levels of calcium inside of brain cells becomes unregulated affecting nerve cell communication and survival.

Other hypotheses: Malfunction of glutamate (NMDA) receptors, herpes virus, neuroinflammatory events, oxidative stress cause the disease.

Table 8.1. A summary of the predominant hypotheses for Alzheimer's disease.

The amyloid and tau hypotheses have been the focus of this book so far, especially in Chapters 6 and 7. They are also the focus of this chapter. In the following chapter we will look at the cholinergic hypothesis. While calling them hypotheses might be a stretch, the importance of NMDA receptors, neuroinflammation and oxidative stress in Alzheimer's disease and its therapies will be covered in subsequent chapters. The link between herpes virus and plaque formation was introduced previously (Chapter 6). The calcium hypothesis which is getting a lot of attention recently will be summarized in Chapter 16.

In spite of all of these hypotheses, in the USA only five drugs have been approved for treatment of Alzheimer's disease. These are discussed in the Chapters 9 and 10. Of these, four are based on cholinesterase (cholinergic hypothesis) and one on the importance of NMDA receptors. In Chapter 14 the complexity that underlies getting to a drug to clinical trial will be discussed which will help to explain why so few drugs have been approved for the treatment of the symptoms associated with Alzheimer's disease.

This chapter will focus on the current research that is being done on plaques and tangles in the hopes of finding drugs that will offer a cure or, more realistically, ways to slow or stop the progression of Alzheimer's disease. To be up front, the number of routes that are being followed is extremely complex. This is because human cells are extremely complicated structures with tens of thousands of proteins doing multiple, cell-specific jobs. Also many pathways that are essential for one job interconnect with other routes that are used to do other things necessary for cell survival and function. To put it another way, while a drug might be used to affect a protein linked to a bad process, at the same time that protein may be needed for other critical, normal cell functions. Often, too, drugs are not 100% specific to a certain protein or other cell target.

Let's look at an example that we are exposed to every day of our lives if we watch television, read magazines or travel the World Wide Web. That topic is erectile deficiency drugs. These drugs are designed to inhibit a very specific enzyme, a protein linked to blood vessel dilation. The trouble is the drug is not as specific as it might be and there are many forms of the enzyme that do other essential jobs in the body that are also affected by the drug. Thus when a certain version of the erectile deficiency drug is taken by certain people, it not only does the intended job but also can affect their vision, increase their heart rate and cause severe headaches among other things.

So with this in mind, in this chapter we will begin by looking at pharmaceutical targets that are linked to the classic hallmarks (plaques and tangles) of Alzheimer's disease first defined by Alois Alzheimer. In the next chapter, we will move on to other hopeful targets. In total we will end by having a relatively complete view of the research that is being done to stop and slow the progression of Alzheimer's disease. While certain drugs and therapies will be mentioned, it is important to remember that this is a dynamic area. At any moment an ongoing study may be terminated for a diversity of reasons. So it is impossible to recommend specific drugs or therapies. This should be done in consultation with biomedical professionals. For the latest information on any specific Alzheimer's drug, the reader should go to one or more websites run by an official Alzheimer's disease society. These are listed at the end of the reference section in this book. There, information on specific drugs, drug trials as well as the latest findings will be covered, usually in a way that the average person will understand.

The Yin-Yang of Plaque Formation as a Target

As detailed in Chapter 6, amyloid beta-containing plaques are widely considered by experts to be a primary distinction of Alzheimer's disease. Amyloid plaque formation is also believed by many to be a central cause of the neurodegenerative events underlying the pathogenesis of Alzheimer's disease. The amyloid beta peptide component of the plaques is produced by the sequential action of two enzymes on the large amyloid precursor protein. The two critical enzymes involved in the formation of amyloid beta peptides are beta-secretase and gamma-secretase. Thus it comes as no surprise that these are also primary targets that have been the focus of research by a number of pharmaceutical companies. The study of amyloid plaque formation for the experimental treatment of Alzheimer's disease started early in the last decade. These lines of research have focused on four main approaches: preventing the formation of the units of plaque formation (amyloid beta peptides), clearance of existing amyloid beta peptides, preventing their aggregation to form amyloid plaques and enhancing the breakdown of existing plaques (Table 8.2).

**Drug Therapies Based
on the
Amyloid Hypothesis**

Decrease amyloid beta formation
Remove existing amyloid beta peptides
Stop amyloid beta aggregation
Remove existing plaques

Table 8.2. Drug therapies based on the amyloid hypothesis.

The amyloid hypothesis still remains a dominant force in understanding how Alzheimer's disease develops. As a result, much translational research has concentrated on the development of therapeutic strategies based on this model. The amyloid hypothesis considers amyloid beta peptide (especially Aβ42) to be the initiator of a pathological cascade that leads to the neurological changes that underlie the onset and progression of the disease, the most common form of dementia in aged adults. Since beta- and gamma-secretase are involved in amyloid beta production, they have become central targets for drug development.

It is important to note that while gamma-secretase is part of the enzymatic sequence that generates amyloid beta, it also cleaves over 24 other proteins. These other functions of gamma-secretase are critical to everyday life functions such as cell adhesion, gene regulation, cell movement and cell communication. Thus while it is difficult to make this enzyme a viable target for intervention, some gamma-secretase inhibitors and modulators are being evaluated (see Table 8.4). Here we will focus primarily on the more promising beta-secretase as a therapeutic target.

We can put all of this information, and a bit more, into the sequence of events leading from amyloid precursor protein (APP) through amyloid beta to plaque formation as shown in Figure 8.1.

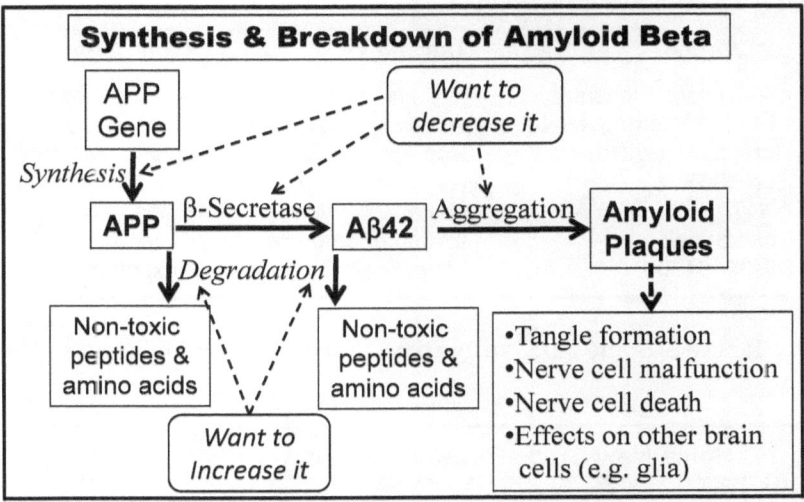

Figure 8.1. Putting amyloid-based drug therapy approaches into context.

Since amyloid precursor protein is the precursor of amyloid beta, some research is aimed at stopping the activity of the gene or the synthesis of the protein as summarized at the end of this chapter. As covered in the previous paragraphs, research is also aimed at decreasing beta-secretase activity and the subsequent aggregation of the amyloid beta peptides into amyloid plaques. In contrast, efforts are underway to increase the degradation of amyloid precursor protein and amyloid beta itself to lower the level of the toxic peptides that lead to plaque formation.

Amyloid Hypothesis-Based Drugs

Clearly there are many approaches being used to deal with amyloid beta production and its transformation into amyloid plaques. Table 8.3 lists some of the past drugs based on the amyloid hypothesis that have failed in trials while table 8.4 lists some of the new drugs that are being evaluated. While many therapeutic approaches have been and are being pursued, here we will focus on beta-secretase to see the reasoning behind them.

Some Failed Drugs Based on the Amyloid Hypothesis		
Drug	Target	Company
r-flurbiprofin/Flurizan®	Reduce Aβ levels	Myriad Genetics
LY450139/semagacestat	γ-/β-secretase inhibitor	Eli Lily & Co.
Homotaurine/Alzhemed™	Stop Aβ aggregation	Neurochem Inc.
ELND006	γ-secretase inhibitor	Elan Corp.
AN1792	Aβ immunotherapy	Elan Corp.
Ponezumab	Aβ immunotherapy	Pfizer Inc.
PF-04494700	Protect cells against Aβ	Pfizer Inc.

Table 8.3. Some failed drugs based on the amyloid hypothesis.

Some New Drugs Based on the Amyloid Hypothesis		
Drug	Target	Company
CTS-21166	β-secretase inhibitor	CoMentis, Inc.
MK-8931	β-secretase inhibitor	Merck & Co.
LY2811376	β-secretase inhibitor	Eli Lilly
TAK-070	β-secretase inhibitor	Takeda Pharm. Co.
Avagacestat	γ-secretase inhibitor	Bristol-Myers/Squib
EVP-0962	γ-secretase modulator	EnVivo Pharmaceuticals
PBT2	β-amyloid aggregation	Prana Biotechnology Ltd.
ELND005	β-amyloid aggregation	Elan Corporation

Table 8.4. Some new drugs based on the amyloid hypothesis.

Let's set the stage for this kind of research by first reviewing amyloid processing which was covered in more detail in Chapter 6. As shown in Figure 8.2, when amyloid precursor protein (APP) is first digested by the enzyme beta-secretase it releases a soluble form of APP (sAPPβ) plus a C-terminal fragment (CTFβ). The membrane-bound CTFβ is then acted on by the second enzyme gamma-secretase which releases amyloid beta (Aβ) plus an intracellular C-terminal fragment (CTFγ). As we know, the amyloid beta that is produced now can serve as a pool of peptide for making amyloid plaques.

On the other hand, the enzyme alpha-secretase mediates the non-amyloidogenic pathway mentioned at the end of the subsection "FYI: The Pathways Leading to Amyloid Beta" in Chapter 6. Alpha-secretase is the natural and more common pathway. It is important in everyday life functions, especially in learning and memory. When alpha-secretase acts on APP, it produces different protein fragments: alpha forms of soluble amyloid precursor protein (sAPPα) and a C-terminal fragment (CTFα) that does not lead to amyloid beta formation. When gamma-secretase then cleaves CTFα it releases a non-amyloidogenic peptide (PS) plus CTFγ.

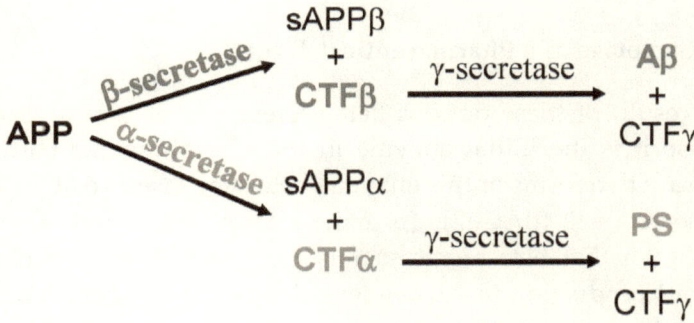

Figure 8.2. The initial cleavage of APP by beta-secretase leads to amyloid beta (Aβ) while cleavage by alpha-secretase does not.

As we can see, there is a Yin-Yang scenario in operation: the production of deadly versus beneficial amyloid peptides depends on whether beta- or alpha-secretase comes into play before gamma-secretase. Since biomedical researchers are interested in reducing amyloid peptide load, then this can be accomplished in different ways as summarized in Figure 8.3. It can be done by decreasing the activity of beta-secretase which will directly decrease amyloid beta formation. Alternatively, it can be done by increasing the activity of alpha-secretase which will stop amyloid peptide formation. In either case, the amount of amyloid beta will be decreased which in turn will decrease the amount of amyloid plaque formation. In theory it is also possible to decrease beta-secretase while increasing alpha-secretase to have an even greater effect at reducing amyloid beta formation. Of course, inhibiting an enzyme like alpha-secretase that has normal cellular functions can lead to unwanted side effects.

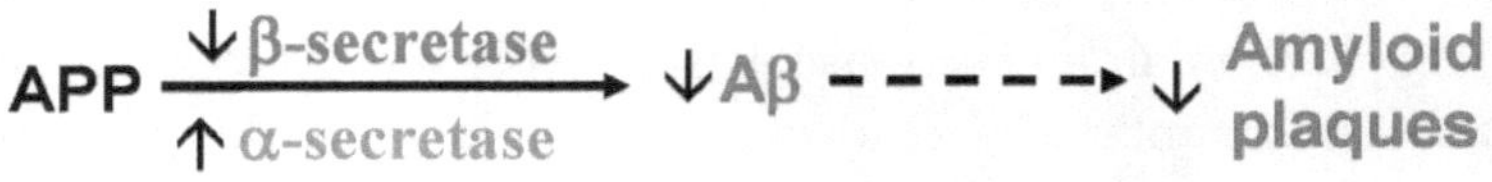

$$\textbf{APP} \xrightarrow[\uparrow \alpha\text{-secretase}]{\downarrow \beta\text{-secretase}} \downarrow A\beta \ -----\dashrightarrow \ \downarrow \ \textbf{Amyloid plaques}$$

Figure 8.3. Altering the way APP is processed by either decreasing beta-secretase activity or increasing alpha-secretase activity leads to reduced amyloid beta formation and potentially reduced production of amyloid plaques.

Beta-Secretase as a Pharmaceutical Target

As a result, of these options beta-secretase is of central interest because it is the initial enzyme in the amyloidogenic pathway. There are two forms of this enzyme, beta-secretase 1 (BACE1) and beta-secretase 2 (BACE2). To make a long story short, research has shown that beta-secretase 1 is likely solely responsible for amyloid production in Alzheimer's disease. While beta-secretase 1 remains a primary target of research, some work has demonstrated that the enzyme might be needed for normal life functions. For example, beta-secretase knockout mice suffer from cognitive defects and other neurological problems. These results suggest that while beta-secretase remains a viable primary target for drug intervention, the goal should be to find agents that reduce but not eliminate this enzyme activity because it does have normal functions. To this end, researchers have generated beta-secretase mutant mice which have only about 50% of the normal level of beta-secretase activity. That work showed that simply reducing beta-secretase activity led to reduced amyloid beta levels as expected. More importantly, those mice showed significantly reduced amyloid plaque formation and synaptic pathologies. As a result, reducing beta-secretase continues to serve as an important and viable target for pharmaceutical intervention.

In addition, some lines of research are aimed at preventing the genes that encode beta-secretase from being activated in humans so that the enzyme will not be synthesized. However, as the mouse studies reveal, complete inhibition of beta-secretase gene activity would not be helpful. It will be interesting to see where those studies end up.

The Continuing Search for Secretase Inhibitors

Since beta-secretase 1 was revealed as the critical secretase involved in amyloid beta production in Alzheimer's disease over a dozen years ago, a great deal of research has been done. Much of the focus has been on developing and testing beta-secretase inhibitors in very early-stage trials. As a result, a large number of inhibitors have been developed and aggressively pursued as pharmaceuticals to combat Alzheimer's disease in many drug trials. Sadly, the nomenclature for these drugs is not designed for easy reading. The first beta-secretase inhibitor that was developed was called P10-P4′ Stat Val (Elan Pharmaceuticals). This drug is part of family of drugs classified as being of the statine type.

Statine is an unusual type of amino acid (4-amino-3-hydroxy-6-methylheptanoic acid). It was discovered as one of the six amino acids that make up pepstatin, a potent inhibitor of certain types of protein-digesting enzymes in our bodies. Because this amino acid is very stable it is used in developing certain types of drugs so that they don't break down quickly. A number of statine-based variants that can be used to inhibit beta-secretase have been synthesized by various companies.

The trouble is, while many early drugs worked great in the test tube, they suffered from a number of characteristics that made them poor pharmaceuticals: they are big molecules, they broke down quickly, they were not useful when taken orally and they had trouble crossing the blood–brain barrier. This explains why they could not be used in human drug trials. However, that early work guided future work and set the stage for the development of other smaller, more effective molecules. One of these is called CTS-21166 (Comentis, Inc.).

In initial human (Phase I) studies, the beta-secretase inhibitor CTS-21166 was found to be safe when injected intravenously. It also reduced the levels of amyloid beta in the blood over an extended period of time. Large amounts of money coupled with partnerships have set the stage for Phase III trials to commence soon. As a result, many international teams of researchers have been working to develop new beta-secretase drugs.

Will New Beta-Secretase Inhibitors Ride to the Rescue?

There is another reason that early studies on beta-secretase inhibitors may have been ineffective at reducing amyloid beta levels and plaque formation in early screening. That reason is the structure of the inhibitors themselves. Apparently previous molecules were too flexible. Like trying to stick a rubber key rather than a metal one into a keyhole, these flexible molecules were not 100% effective. This problem is apparently no longer an issue, as the recent patent list (2006–2011) of beta-secretase inhibitors attests. In the works is a long list of small molecule inhibitors that some suggest will solve previous problems and lead to effective drugs to reduce plaque load. It is hoped these drugs will at least reduce if not stop the progression of the disease. These molecules fall into a diversity of categories based on their mode of action and biochemical attributes. For example there are statine-type variants like P10-P4' Stat Val discussed above. As well, there are a diversity of others with names that would make a chemist drool but make the rest of us shake our heads: various variations of amines, hydroxyethylamines, arylamino compounds and hydantoins, to name a few. However, it is unlikely we'll see any of these in human clinical trials or on the market for many years to come.

There are other routes that might offer more rapid progress but are not in the headlights of mainstream pharmaceutical companies. For example, recently enzyme studies in vitro showed for the first time that beta-secretase 1 activity is increased by calcium levels as well as by calmodulin, a primary calcium sensor protein in all cells. Furthermore, antagonists of calmodulin reduced beta-secretase 1 activity by at least 50%, thus fitting with a level consistent and appropriate for pharmaceutical intervention as suggested by data discussed in the previous paragraph.

Considering the central role of calcium in models of Alzheimer's disease (Table 8.1; Chapter 16), these results should be considered as potential therapeutic routes. More to the point, a number of antagonists of calmodulin exist that have already been shown to be harmless in humans. This is just one example of the routes that can be taken as the search for an effective Alzheimer's therapy continues. In the meantime a great deal of effort and money is being expended to find effective and useful beta-secretase inhibitors. Now, let's look at therapies surrounding the second primary hallmark of Alzheimer's disease, neurofibrillary tangles.

Treatments Targeting Tau

As might be expected from what has been covered throughout this volume, many developing therapies are based on the protein tau, the culprit in forming neurofibrillary tangles. In Chapter 7, we saw the events that transform normal, essential tau into its demonic phosphorylated form that makes up neurofibrillary tangles. We have also learned that the amount of tangle formation in Alzheimer's brain regions is directly related to the amount of observed cognitive decline. Thus, targeting the stages from tau modification to tangle formation is of prime interest. Thus the first stage in making good tau bad is the addition of phosphate groups (phosphorylation). In fact, a large number of phosphate groups are progressively added to tau so it is said to be hyperphosphorylated. One approach that researchers are using involves preventing the addition of phosphate groups to tau proteins. Let's look at a revised figure of one we first saw in Chapter 7 to understand this (Figure 8.4).

Enzymes that add phosphate groups to molecules are called kinases (Figure 8.4). Progressive phosphorylation of tau converts it to P-tau, which organizes in a series of steps into the neurofibrillary tangles of the Alzheimer's brain. Inside neurons are enzymes called phosphatases that remove the phosphate groups from P-tau. These phosphatases thus convert it back to unphosphorylated tau.

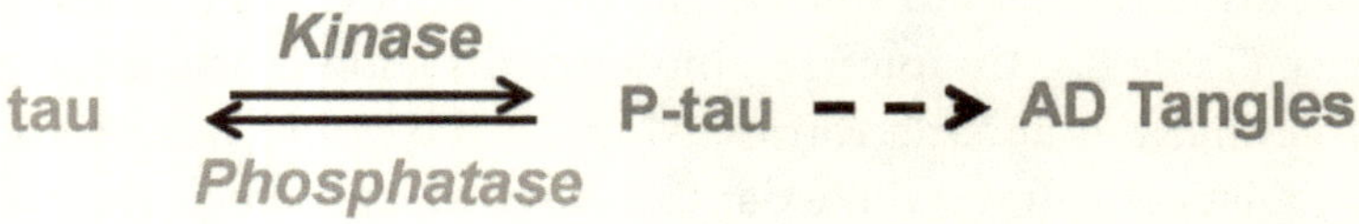

Kinase

tau ⇌ **P-tau – – ➤ AD Tangles**

Phosphatase

Figure 8.4. Tau is phosphorylated by kinases to produce P-tau,
the major component of Alzheimer's disease tangles.
P-tau can be dephosphorylated by phosphatase activity.

The following simple diagram reveals two clear routes to stopping or at least slowing tangle formation (Figure 8.5). The first is to inhibit the kinase activity so tau doesn't get phosphorylated. The second is to stimulate or enhance phosphatase activity so any phosphorylated tau is quickly dephosphorylated. Let's put some names to these enzymes and see just what is being done to put this theoretical model into practice.

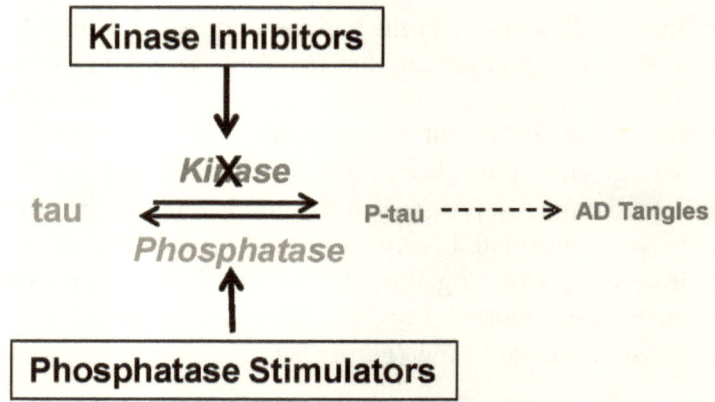

Figure 8.5. The inhibition of kinase activity or enhancement of
phosphatase activity can lead to reduced phosphorylated tau
and reduced tangle formation.

Many Kinases Turn Good Tau Bad

While there are many different kinases in our bodies that can add phosphate groups to a diversity of proteins, only one kinase is believed to the major one that adds phosphate groups to tau proteins. It is called glycogen synthase kinase 3 (GSK3) because it also plays a role in glycogen metabolism. Like many cell proteins, GSK3 serves many functions but its deadly role involves the hyperphosphorylation of tau. Because a lot of pure, non-medical research has been done in a diversity of animals a lot is known about GSK3 and various inhibitors of the enzyme have been developed or discovered.

One inhibitor of GSK3 is lithium chloride (LiCl), a mood-stabilizing drug. Lithium is used to treat bipolar disorder so it already has a pharmacological history. Lithium is an element (Li) found on the periodic table. Lithium salts have a long history for use in people with bipolar disorder. Lithium also stabilizes mood and is sometimes used for the treatment of depression and mania. It has been proven to reduce tau phosphorylation and tangle formation in mice and is currently being studied for human use. It is somewhat effective but it also affects other things, so it's not the best solution to preventing tau hyperphosphorylation. Several other inhibitors of GSK3 (e.g., CHIR-98014, SB216763, SRN-003-556) are also currently being evaluated for use in Alzheimer's therapies.

A number of drugs have been developed that inhibit CDK5, another kinase involved in the phosphorylation of tau. CDK5 is present in high levels in the brain. Existing CDK5 drugs also have side effects due in part to the fact that CDK5 has multiple essential functions, including regulating neurogenesis (formation and growth of nerve cells). Also, while there are many CDK5 inhibitors in existence, few have been used outside of primary research. In short, for the most part they have been used to treat cells in culture but not whole animals or humans.

Drugs that Prevent or Reduce Tangles

While much research is aimed at stopping the phosphorylation of tau, other approaches have also been taken to reduce the formation of tangles in the Alzheimer's brain. Drugs have been developed that stop the toxic aggregation of hyperphosphorylated tau proteins, the initial step towards full-fledged tangle formation. Interestingly, methylene blue, a dye that is used to identify tangles in post-mortem brain sections, has successfully moved from Phase II to Phase III clinical trials. Other drugs (e.g., anthraquinones) that also affect tau aggregation have been developed and are being tested in animal models. Related to this is research for finding ways to make hyperphosphorylated tau break down so that is unavailable for tangle formation. Protein breakdown in cells is a complex event that occurs via a number or pathways. That said, one approach is to inhibit a protein called heat shock protein 90 which protects phosphorylated tau from degradation. An inhibitor of this enzyme (EC102) was effective at reducing the amount of hyperphosphorylated tau in mouse brains as well as in homogenates of Alzheimer's brains. The stage is now set to translate this initial biomedical research into an effective therapy for Phase II and III testing.

Why Do Some Promising Drugs Fail?

The lack of efficacy of many of the currently used pharmaceuticals may not always be due to the fact that they are ineffective. It more likely has to do with the fact that the drug is being applied too late. In other words, by the time amyloid beta begins to appear and accumulate in plaques, the seeds of cognitive decline may already be set in motion—possibly with an unstoppable, irreversible momentum. For this reason, one area of focus is to determine exactly when these seeds of destruction are sown. What is the initial event that starts the progression towards plaque formation? One research area is on detecting biomarkers that signal the earliest events in the stage of Alzheimer's disease, as detailed in Chapter 11. In terms of amyloid accumulation, for example, the presence of altered levels of amyloid beta peptide in cerebrospinal fluid is one biomarker that is under evaluation. With knowledge of when this peptide first appears in the wrong places, drug therapy could be initiated to stop its transformation into harmful plaques.

Chapter 9

Targeting the Cholinergic Hypothesis

As indicated in Table 8.1 in the previous chapter, the cholinergic hypothesis is one of the central hypotheses of Alzheimer's disease. It is considered to be the oldest of all the models attempting to explain the causes and effects of the disease. It is based upon acetylcholine, the first known neurotransmitter. In Alzheimer's disease, the levels of acetylcholine and numbers of receptors for it drop. It has been estimated that there is a loss of between 40–70% of neurons that use this transmitter in the brains of those with Alzheimer's disease. So the goals of research have been to re-establish the cholinergic neuron population and/or the functional levels of acetylcholine, allowing them to function more like they do in the normal brain.

The Cholinergic Hypothesis

In Chapter 5 we summarized the general events of neuron function and the role of neurotransmitters. Here we will re-examine neurotransmission by focusing on acetylcholine specifically. This will also set the stage for our examination of NMDA receptors and Alzheimer's disease in the following chapter. In doing so we'll understand more fully the primary way brain nerve cells talk to each other — how messages are passed from one nerve cell to the next in the brain. This information is critical for the understanding of drug therapies that are currently in use as well as those that are being developed.

Of central interest in Alzheimer's disease are the "cholinergic neurons". These neurons communicate with each other using acetylcholine (Figure 9.1). If we consider two nerve cells, the first nerve cell makes and secretes this chemical while the second cell binds to it and converts the chemical signal to a cellular response. Acetylcholine is called a neurotransmitter because it can transmit messages between neurons. It can also transmit messages from a nerve cell to a muscle cell. In fact this is how our skeletal muscles are controlled, by nerve cells that release acetylcholine. Acetylcholine is also involved in regulating stomach muscle contraction and enzyme secretion from the pancreas, among other roles. So this chemical is a very common and central molecule of communication throughout our bodies. In the brain, acetylcholine regulates a person's attention, working memory and other cognitive functions.

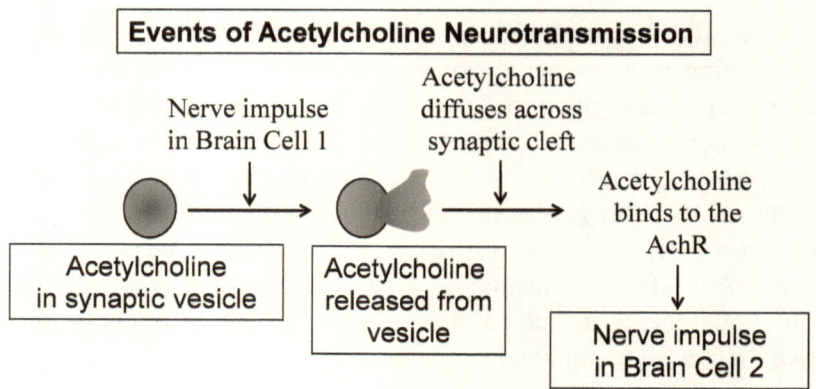

Figure 9.1. Acetylcholine as a neurotransmitter.
AchR, acetylcholine receptor.

The events of acetylcholine neurotransmission are summarized in Figure 9.1. This is essentially the same figure as Figure 5.9 that was presented in Chapter 5 except it is revised for acetylcholine. Thus, acetylcholine molecules (Figure 9.2) that are present in synaptic vesicles are released from one neuron in response to a nerve impulse. They diffuse across the synapse where they bind to acetylcholine receptors (AchR), setting up a nerve impulse in the next neuron.

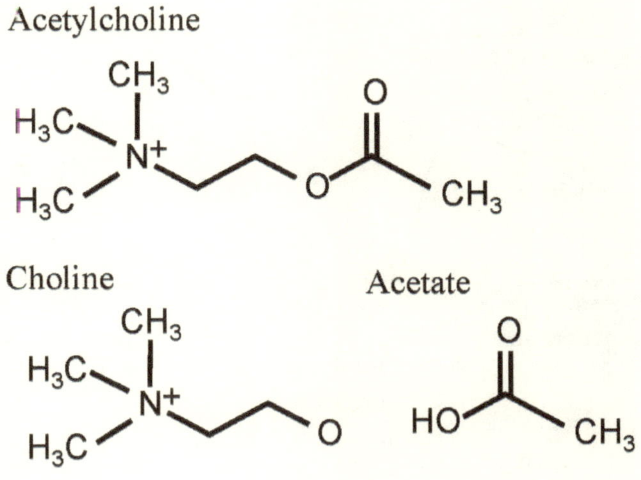

Acetylcholine

Choline   Acetate

Figure 9.2. Structure of acetylcholine, choline and acetate.

In Alzheimer's individuals the function of acetylcholine neurons is impaired. Early on, this knowledge led to the development of the "Cholinergic Hypothesis" of Alzheimer's disease. Post-mortem analyses of Alzheimer's brains have shown that the amount of acetylcholine produced by neurons is decreased. In addition, the amount of this chemical that is released is also significantly decreased. As if this weren't enough, the ability to receive the acetylcholine message is decreased because there are fewer receptors to bind to it. Thus in our two-nerve-cell system, the first cell makes too little and then releases even less acetylcholine while the second nerve cell is barely able to understand what little message has been sent.

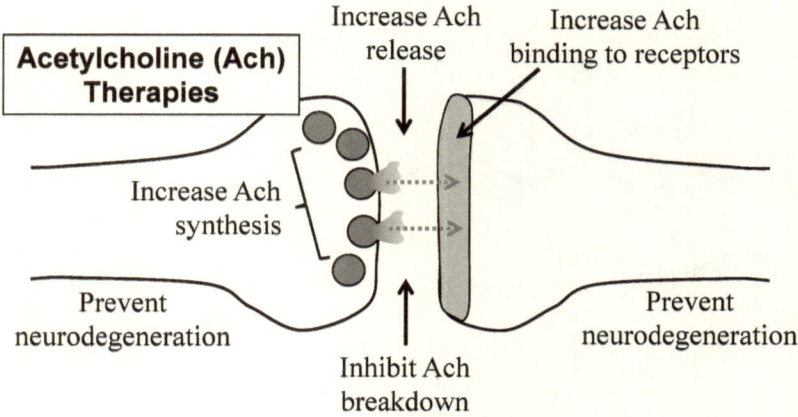

Figure 9.3. Some goals of acetylcholine therapies.

Therapies Based on Acetylcholine

There are several approaches based on acetylcholine communication that are being taken to stop neurodegeneration. These are summarized in Figure 9.3. Enhancing the synthesis of acetylcholine can be used to make up for decreasing levels of the neurotransmitter in Alzheimer's neurons. Similarly, increasing the rate of acetylcholine release into synapses would be beneficial. Inhibition of acetylcholinesterase, to prevent acetylcholine breakdown, is an easier and often exploited approach. Finally, increasing the amount of binding of acetylcholine to its receptor and/or increasing the number of receptors would help in alleviating the decreased levels of the neurotransmitter in the Alzheimer's brain.

* * *

FYI: More about Acetylcholine Receptors

Some nerve cells release acetylcholine and others bind to it and respond appropriately. To respond to acetylcholine the cell must have a receptor for it. While it doesn't tell the whole story, it's like a lock and key—acetylcholine, the key, binds to its receptor, the lock, to open the door to a specific cellular response. Drugs are being developed to affect acetylcholine, its receptor and the signaling events that are initiated by their interaction in the brain. So let's look specifically at acetylcholine brain receptors that are linked to memory: muscarinic acetylcholine receptors.

Muscarinic acetylcholine receptors bind to acetylcholine (Ach) to mediate downstream signaling events in various cells, tissues and organs. Their name derives from the fact they are more sensitive to a chemical called muscarine. (Many of the pharmaceuticals in use today originated from naturally occurring biological molecules.) Muscarine is a poisonous agent produced by certain types of mushrooms. There are five different muscarinic acetylcholine receptors: M1–5. Of these, M1 is involved in memory. The green mamba snake from Africa has been a kind donor of several specific inhibitors of mAch receptors. The deadly venom from this large snake has been shown to contain three polypeptides that are specific for the mAchR inhibitors M1, M2 and M4. These snake venom inhibitors have assisted in the dissection of the intracellular events mediated by these receptors.

Figure 9.4 presents a basic diagram to explain this. Acetylcholine binds to an M1 muscarinic acetylcholine receptor causing it, in turn, to activate a signaling complex in the nerve cell membrane. Through a sequence of events, the calcium levels increase inside the cell. When properly stimulated, the levels of calcium inside the cell allow the nerves to operate normally. When calcium levels are not properly controlled they affect neuron function. This is the basis of the "Calcium Hypothesis" of Alzheimer's disease.

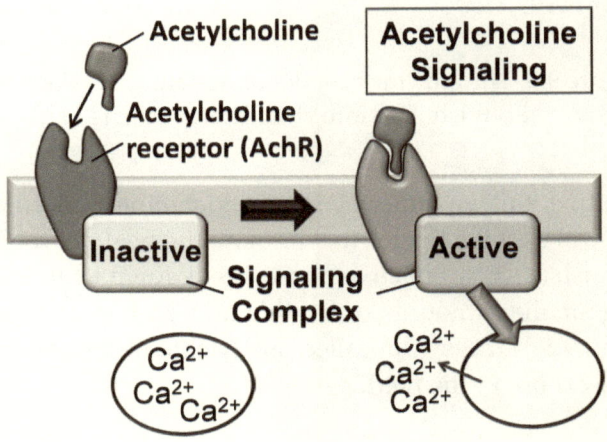

Figure 9.4. Acetylcholine (Ach) binds to a receptor (mAchR), ultimately causing calcium to be released within nerve cells.

* * *

Acetylcholinesterase Inhibitors

So a number of approaches have been developed to improve the communication between acetylcholine-based neurons in people with Alzheimer's disease. One approach is to increase the levels of acetylcholine that survive once the chemical is released. This is needed because even in normal neurons there is an enzyme called acetylcholinesterase that breaks down any released acetylcholine. As shown in Figure 9.5, the enzyme converts acetylcholine to choline and acetate. While acetylcholinesterase activity actually decreases at synapses in the Alzheimer's brain, there is still plenty present to remove existing acetylcholine. In contrast, high levels of acetylcholinesterase are associated with amyloid plaques. There is research data showing that this enzyme is involved in amyloid beta fiber formation. Thus, this is another reason for reducing the levels of acetylcholinesterase activity in the Alzheimer's brain. In theory, inhibiting acetylcholinesterase would allow more acetylcholine to survive permitting this communication to occur relatively normally. It could also stop or slow plaque formation.

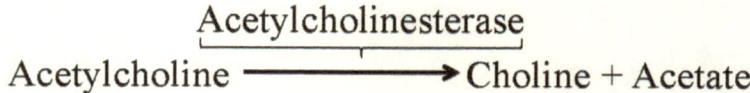

Figure 9.5. The enzyme acetylcholinesterase breaks down acetylcholine into choline and acetate.

By inhibiting this enzyme, every acetylcholine molecule that is released will survive longer to stimulate the next nerve. Since the inhibitor isn't 100% effective some breakdown still will occur, releasing smaller amounts of choline and acetate as represented in Figure 9.6. Drugs are called acetylcholinesterase inhibitors (AchEI) by those in the field.

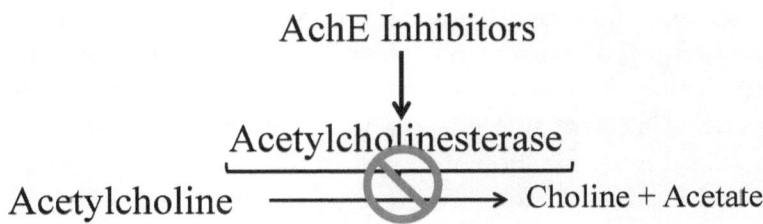

Figure 9.6. AchE inhibitors inhibit the enzyme acetylcholinesterase, stopping or slowing the breakdown of acetylcholine into choline and acetate (as suggested by their decreased font size).

FDA-Approved Cholinergic Drugs

This, in fact, has become the primary therapeutic approach to controlling the cognitive loss associated with Alzheimer's disease as well as other forms of dementia. Those acetylcholinesterase pharmaceuticals that have been approved by the FDA in the US are listed in Table 9.1. Over the past three decades, the drug tacrine has been useful in treating the symptoms of Alzheimer's disease. Tacrine is rarely prescribed today because of its serious side effects. More recently three other acetylcholinesterase drugs, donepezil, galantamine and rivastigmine, have been approved for use. While the prevention of memory loss and other cognitive defects has been subtle, it has been shown that acetylcholinesterase drug therapy is still the most effective with the least serious side effects. That said, the drugs are not effective for everyone, likely since the underlying causes and symptoms of Alzheimer's disease vary widely from person to person. Finally, the side effects of these drugs can include nausea, vomiting, diarrhea and tremors. More to the point, the drugs don't protect nerve cells over time nor do they prevent the outcome of the disease.

So these pharmaceuticals are recommended for alleviating the symptoms of Alzheimer's disease; they do not provide a cure nor do they stop its progression. In light of this, the following are some general comments that should be considered but are not meant to define how treatment should be carried out or its success evaluated. Due to side effects some have suggested appropriate doses for these drugs: donepezil (10 mg), galantamine (24 mg) and rivastigmine (12 mg). For the rivastigmine patch, 9.2 mg is recommended. These drugs should never be administered without a long-term follow-up plan of defined treatment goals set up by your doctor. Patient monitoring should be done regularly. Any significant adverse side effects should be noted and, if serious, could lead to termination of the use of the drug. Success needs to be evaluated with cognitive testing to verify if there is any improvement or, at worst, not decreasing. This is usually done by three to six months after starting the therapy.

Five FDA-Approved Alzheimer's Drugs

Drug	Category	Stage	Side Effects
Donepezil (Aricept)	Cholinesterase inhibitor	All stages	Nausea, vomiting, loss of appetite, increased bowel movements
Glantamine (Razadyne)	Cholinesterase inhibitor	Mild to Moderate	Nausea, vomiting, loss of appetite, increased bowel movements
Rivastigmine (Exelon)	Cholinesterase inhibitor	Mild to Moderate	Nausea, vomiting, loss of appetite, increased bowel movements
Tacrine (Cognex)	Cholinesterase inhibitor	Mild to Moderate	Nausea, vomiting, liver damage possible (rarely prescribed)
Memantine	NMDA receptor	Moderate to Severe	Headache, constipation, confusion, dizziness

Table 9.1. Five FDA-approved Alzheimer's drugs. "Cholinesterase" is used here for "acetylcholinesterase" since it is often referred to this way. Memantine is the only non-acetylcholinesterase pharmaceutical.

As we have mentioned many times, any drug can have multiple effects in the body. When an inhibitor of acetylcholinesterase is ingested it enters the bloodstream, ultimately affecting all tissues. Acetylcholine is not only important in communication between nerves, it has many other functions. In the pancreas, acetylcholine affects the two primary cell types of this organ differently. It causes pancreatic acinar cells to secrete digestive enzymes, including amylase and trypsinogen. On the other hand, it affects the beta cells of the pancreas to secrete insulin. The parotid (salivary) glands are also affected by acetylcholine which stimulates the release of amylase. Acetylcholine also affects events other than secretion in non-nerve cells because it regulates smooth muscle contraction in the stomach. Thus while the low levels of acetylcholine in the Alzheimer's brain will be augmented by inhibitors of acetylcholinesterase, other tissues can be harmed. This is because these inhibitors can lead to an increase in acetylcholine beyond what is normally required in these cells, which could lead to enhanced enzyme secretion by pancreatic acinar cells and the parotid glands. It could also mean increased insulin release as well as enhanced stimulation of stomach muscle contraction. This might explain some of the side effects associated with acetylcholinesterase inhibitors listed in Table 9.1.

Clinical Variations Can Hide Information

One of the issues facing any drug study is variability. Thus while a drug may not pan out statistically on a population-wide scale, there is still the possibility that a specific drug might work on a subset of individuals. This is why pharmaceutical studies are being redesigned on a regular basis to determine if a drug might benefit a smaller group of individuals rather than everyone. This is dealt with in more detail in Chapter 14. So let's look at some aspects of this problem in terms of acetylcholinesterase inhibitors.

During the decades that acetylcholinesterase inhibitors have been in use, clinicians have developed a diversity of unique protocols for administering acetylcholinesterase inhibitor drugs without paying attention to how others have done their studies. Some of these variations are summarized in Table 9.2 and detailed here.

Early Drug Study Variability

❖ Different cholinesterase drugs used
❖ Variation in how drug was given
❖ Difference in amount given
❖ Difference in number of treatments
❖ Variation in stage when drug given
❖ Success assessment methods vary

Table 9.2. A list of reasons for variability in the results from different drug studies.

Not only does this variability confound researchers attempting to validate a drug's efficacy but it also means that some less-than-optimal protocols have been used by some clinicians, making their data useless. This means some data cannot be used in what is called meta-analysis research. These are data-mining studies which compile results from a diversity of other studies to find statistically significant results which may have been undetected in the individual studies. For example, variations in therapy have included how the drug is administered (oral versus transdermal patch), the amount administered, when the drug was administered and the length of time it was administered. The stage of the disease when the drug is administered also causes problems in comparing data. So let's look at some of the variations in treatment that exist both in relation to the issue of meta-analysis and for a general understanding of how pharmacotherapy approaches are being evaluated and changed based on early results.

Clearly, starting a drug therapy as soon as possible is the best scenario. However, early memory loss due to Alzheimer's disease is often dismissed as simply due to aging. Thus, most drug therapies start later in the progression of the disease when significant brain changes have already occurred. (The issue of defining when Alzheimer's disease starts or what initiates the disease is discussed several times within the book.) It is known that significant cholinergic deficits don't usually appear until the later stages of brain degeneration; they are minimal in the mild cognitive stages. Thus, should an anti-cholinesterase drug such as donepezil, galantamine or rivastigmine be given before significant changes in cholinergic function appear or after? The results to date suggest that either option has led to some positive results. Treating later stages of Alzheimer's disease can temporarily slow the progress of the disease. On the other hand, by treating early there are potentially greater benefits to the patient by prolonging the mild cognitive impairment phase during which the patient's quality of life is still relatively normal.

Another issue that arises is drug dosage. Because of side effects, some patients get oral drug dosages that are not optimal. Some clinicians believe that using transdermal administration, as is possible with rivastigmine, diminishes some of the side effects caused by oral administration. This also improves the chances of increasing drug dosages so they become more or completely optimal. This is important because it has been argued that early administration of sufficient dosages is the best way to slow the progression of Alzheimer's disease.

The last issue concerns the methods of assessment that were used in drug studies. The way the success of the drug was evaluated varied widely. Some studies used a single test of effectiveness while others used two or more. Some used psychological testing with the type of testing varying from study to study. Others quantified biochemical markers such as amyloid beta levels but the way this was done and the source (e.g., blood vs. cerebrospinal fluid) varied.

All of the above issues are further confounded by the fact that the duration of drug treatment is usually too short. Alzheimer's sufferers and their caregivers traditionally show a low level of compliance with drug therapies. Usually those with the disease only last four to five months on any drug therapy plan, then they drop out of the program. This is often due to having too many medications to take and due to forgetfulness. The transition from giving drugs orally to the use of transdermal patches is seen as a way to improve the length of time those with Alzheimer's disease stay with their respective drug regimen. The issue here is that not all drugs can be administered this way. However, as time goes on, scientists will undoubtedly develop forms of effective drugs that can be administered through the skin. They will also develop drug regimens that are more effective and easier to follow.

So the search continues for more effective and specific acetylcholinesterase inhibitors. Currently around a dozen different drugs are being investigated while many other investigations are focusing on other aspects of the acetylcholine-mediated communication system in brain cells. In the next chapter we will focus on NMDA receptors, which respond to the neurotransmitter glutamate. While there is a progressive loss of functional acetylcholine communication by neurons that therapies try to recover, the situation with NMDA receptors is just the reverse. Therapies are being developed to stop their function.

Chapter 10

NMDA Receptors as Pharmaceutical Targets

NMDA receptors are the second target for which partially effective pharmaceuticals have been developed. After introducing what these receptors are and how they work, the current state of affairs regarding the value of this target in Alzheimer's therapy will be covered.

Glutamate and NMDA Receptors

NMDA receptors (NMDAR) are the receptors for the neurotransmitter glutamate. Glutamate or glutamic acid is the major excitatory neurotransmitter. In fact 70% of all neurons in the central nervous system use glutamate receptors. Being one of the amino acids, it is also the most predominant neurotransmitter in the body. Many have felt the effects, such as dizziness, when they have had food with too much monosodium glutamate in it. This is because this food flavouring agent also binds to glutamate receptors.

There are several types of glutamate receptors that work in different ways. However, here we are interested in one of these: the NMDA receptors. These glutamate receptors are so named because they were identified due to their antagonism by the chemical NMDA (N-methyl-D-aspartate). Like for many topics covered in this book, numerous complete volumes have been written about the NMDA receptors so we will be getting the short and Alzheimer's-specific version. This brings us to the role of NMDA receptors in the Alzheimer's brain.

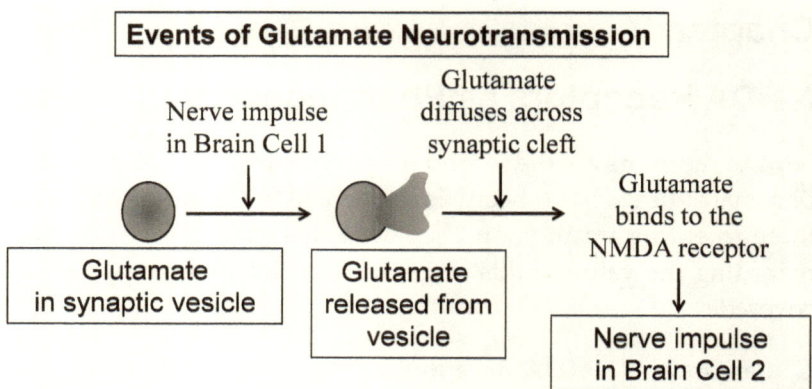

Figure 10.1. Glutamate as a neurotransmitter.

While the names and specific details change, the events of glutamate neurotransmission follow the same basic scheme as detailed previously for acetylcholine neurotransmission (Chapter 9). As summarized in Figure 10.1, glutamate molecules that are present in synaptic vesicles are released from one neuron in response to a nerve impulse. They diffuse across the synapse where they bind to glutamate receptors (NMDA receptors), setting up a nerve impulse in the next neuron.

NMDA Receptors as Pharmacological Targets

The NMDA receptor is an ion channel (Figure 10.2). When the neurotransmitter glutamate is released from synaptic vesicles it diffuses across the synaptic cleft. At the post-synaptic membrane, glutamate binds to the NMDA receptor and the channel opens, allowing sodium ions and calcium ions to flow into the post-synaptic neuron. This sets up an action potential in this neuron.

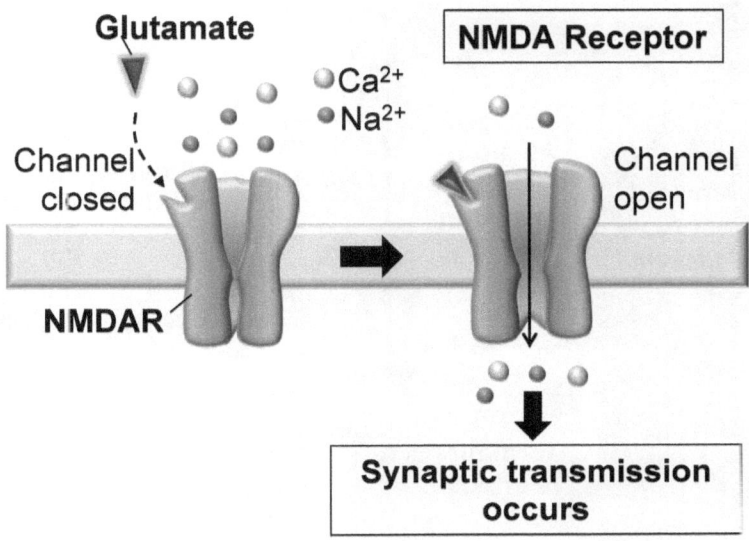

Figure 10.2. Events of glutamate neurotransmission.

NMDA receptors have been a pharmacological target in Alzheimer's disease for a number of reasons but most of all because of their central role in learning and memory. Fitting with this role is the high density of glutamate and specifically NMDA receptors in the hippocampus of the brain. More recently, there is emerging evidence for a central role of NMDA receptors in amyloid beta accumulation and function. This is summarized in Figure 10.3. Some have suggested that the NMDA receptor is also a receptor for amyloid beta, either by directly or indirectly binding to it. Other evidence indicates that NMDA receptors may mediate the actions of amyloid beta on synaptic transmission and plasticity. Two other roles for the NMDA receptor have also been areas of focus: amyloid beta's effect on the function of the NMDA receptor and, vice versa, the receptor's possible control of amyloid beta formation. Any or all of these functions may prove to be true, which provides more arguments for focussing on NMDA receptors as pharmaceutical targets in Alzheimer's disease. Let's look at some specific pharmacological approaches that have been taken. Then we will view some that are in the works or under consideration.

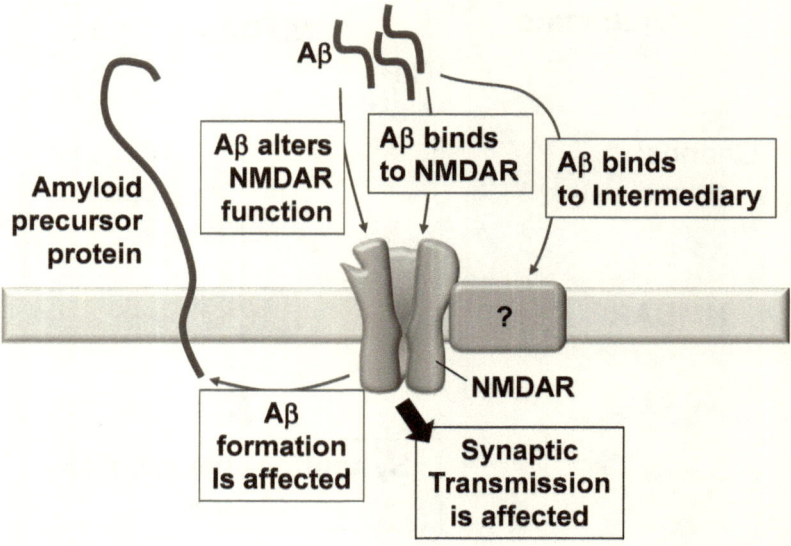

Figure 10.3. The NMDA receptor (NMDAR) is involved in
many aspects of amyloid beta formation and function.
(After Malinow, 2012)

While it is known that neuronal cell death in Alzheimer's brains
leads to excess glutamate release, the situation with glutamate
receptors is less well understood. In spite of the importance
of NMDA receptors in Alzheimer's disease, there is little
information on what exactly happens to these receptors and their
neurons during the early and late stages of the disease. A recent
study was done in an Alzheimer's-like rat model system to
understand what may be occurring. That study showed that
levels of a specific NMDA receptor known as NR2B increased in
the hippocampus in the brains of these "Alzheimer's disease"
rats. This suggests that the events of altered neurotransmission
and neuronal cell death could be due in part to too much of this
NMDA receptor forming in the Alzheimer's brain. These results
also tie in with the main drug being used to target NMDA
receptors of individuals suffering from Alzheimer's disease.

Memantine as an Alzheimer's Drug

There is only one current NMDA receptor antagonist that is being
used clinically for the treatment of Alzheimer's disease. That drug

is memantine. Memantine binds to a specific group of NMDA receptors, preventing ion channel opening. These receptors are of the NR2B type as discussed in the previous paragraph. Memantine doesn't bind to the glutamate-binding site but to other regions of these NMDA receptors. As summarized in Figure 10.4, the binding of memantine prevents the opening of the ion channel receptor, thus stopping the harmful increase in levels of calcium inside these neurons.

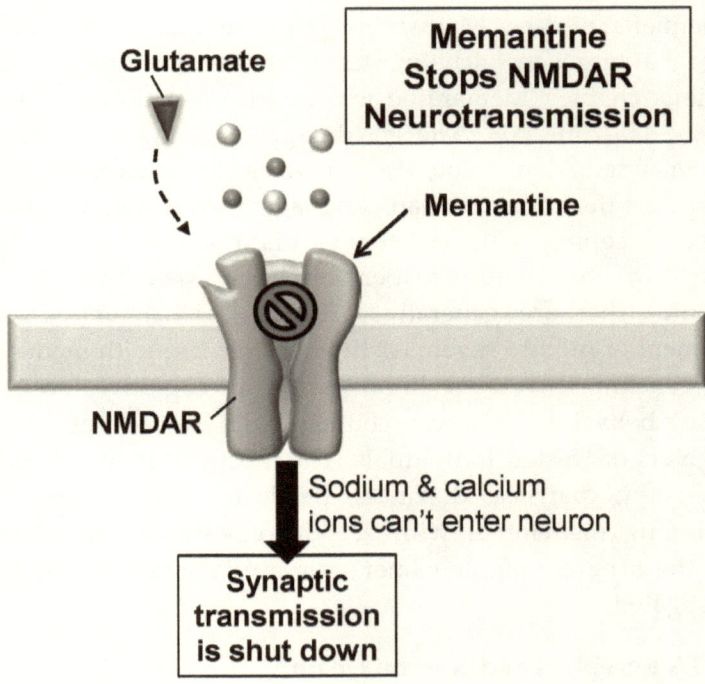

Figure 10.4. Memantine blocks neurotransmission by binding to the NMDA receptor.

There is an extensive literature on the use and effectiveness of memantine. Here we will comment on a few issues. Work with model systems has verified that memantine treatment attenuates the harmful effects of amyloid beta and protects other (e.g., cholinergic) neurons against neuronal cell death. It also prevents the progressive development of memory impairment in rats. Part of this effect might be explained by evidence that memantine reduces the level of tau phosphorylation and, as a result, the accumulation of neurofibrillary tangles. In addition, in human cell lines, memantine appears to increase the alpha-secretase pathway leading to the production of the safe form of soluble amyloid precursor protein and reduced amyloid beta levels. Thus there is evidence that memantine may be effective at many levels in humans as well.

As indicated, memantine is the only drug targeting the NMDA receptor that is approved for use in humans suffering from Alzheimer's disease. Memantine plus the four FDA-approved drugs that target acetylcholinesterase are listed in Table 9.1 in the previous chapter. Memantine was approved in Europe in 2002 and the USA in 2003. A target dosage of 10 mg twice daily is recommended. Memantine, also known as Namenda, is prescribed to improve the attention span, language, memory, and reasoning of people coping with Alzheimer's disease. It is also designed to improve their ability to perform basic tasks. (All these are attributes that are generally lost with Alzheimer's disease.) Treatment of mild to severe Alzheimer's disease with memantine has been linked to some improvement in cognitive levels and general behavior. This was coupled with some relief for the caregivers of treated individuals. The most common side effects are anxiety, diarrhea, dizziness, headaches and hypertension. Combining memantine with acetylcholinesterase inhibitors to slow the progress of Alzheimer's disease is another route being investigated.

NMDA Receptors and Neuron Death

There's another aspect of NMDA receptors that is also central to Alzheimer's disease. When glutamate receptors are stimulated for an extended period of time, this can lead to neurodegeneration. This event is called neurotoxicity. Many independent groups of neuroscientists have linked the disturbance in glutamate neurotransmission with some of the neuropathological events that underlie Alzheimer's disease. As neurons die in the Alzheimer's brain, excess glutamate is released. This unregulated release acts on existing NMDA receptor-containing neurons to over stimulate them. The chronic stimulation of the NMDA receptors results in a neuronal overload of calcium ions. This influx of excess calcium first damages the ability of nerves to function properly by shutting down normal neurotransmission. With continued calcium influx, cell death of neurons is inevitable. These events are in keeping with the calcium hypothesis of Alzheimer's disease that is detailed in Chapter 16.

Chapter 11

Biomarkers: Detecting Alzheimer's Disease

Biomarkers and Their Uses

Biomarkers were introduced in Chapter 1 but were not fully defined or explained. A biomarker, as its name implies, is a biological marker. It is some biological attribute that is objectively measured to determine whether a person's health is normal or if they are suffering from a pathogenic process. Let's be a bit more specific. The biomarkers we've seen so far have been amyloid beta, tau and phospho-tau. We've also mentioned PET, MRI and other brain scans. Psychological testing was also touched upon. In essence these are the three major types of biomarker categories as summarized in Figure 11.1: Biochemical, Brain Imaging and Behavioral. These categories are based on extensive work done by a large number of biomedical researchers.

Types & Examples of AD Biomarkers	
Biomarker	*Example*
Biochemical	Aβ42, tau, p-tau in CSF, etc.
Brain imaging	PET scan, MRI, EEG. etc.
Behavioral	Cognitive, psychological testing

Figure 11.1. The types of biomarkers and examples from Alzheimer's disease. Aβ42, amyloid beta 42; CSF, cerebrospinal fluid; EEG, electroencephalogram; PET, positron emission tomography; MRI, magnetic resonance imaging.

Thus the levels of amyloid beta, tau and phospho-tau in cerebrospinal fluid are indicators of specific stages of Alzheimer's disease and they correlate with specific stages and behavioral changes associated with the disease. These biomarkers are measured using biochemical methods with cerebrospinal fluid, blood and tissue. Brain imaging involves a diversity of techniques (e.g., PET, MRI, EEG) which allow us to assess brain changes in

Alzheimer's individuals. Based on the technique and how it is applied it can provide information not only in terms of active areas of the brain and changes in sizes of various regions, but also in the localization of specific molecules such as amyloid beta. Behavioral changes can be assessed by a diversity of cognitive and other psychological tests (e.g., MMSE, CDR-sb, ADAS-cog) which we will define and comment upon later in this chapter.

Biomarkers have a number of uses which are summarised in Figure 11.2. Various types of biomarkers can be used to assess the status and progress of Alzheimer's disease. This allows doctors to prescribe specific drugs and non-drug therapies to help the individual. Biomarkers also have other uses, especially in finding new therapeutic targets which can guide research into producing appropriate pharmaceuticals. The third value of biomarkers is in their use in evaluating the success of such treatments during clinical trials. The success of specific therapies at each stage of a clinical trial or when an individual is on an already-approved pharmaceutical regimen can be assessed by measuring the status-appropriate biochemical, behavioral or brain imaging biomarkers.

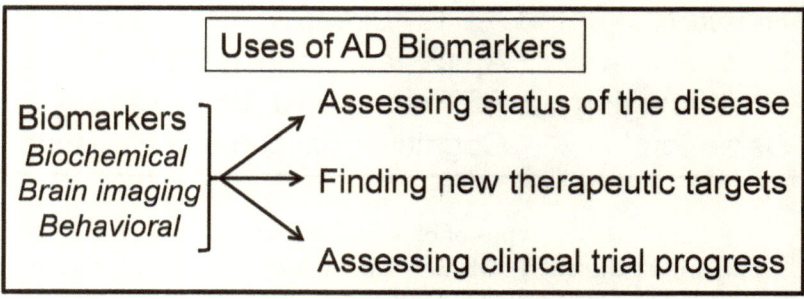

Figure 11.2. The uses of Alzheimer's disease biomarkers.

As scientists continue their search for biomarkers they hopefully will, for lack of a better word, stumble upon new, more precise biomarkers. This is likely how biomarkers linked to the onset of Alzheimer's disease will be discovered — ah, serendipity, you play such a key role in biomedical discoveries! The key to such serendipitous events, however, relies on sound experimental design and knowledge which opens the door to "luck". Alois Alzheimer didn't know what he would find when he dissected the brain of Alzheimer's individuals. But through luck coupled with his expert knowledge, he was able to see that Alzheimer's brains had some novel attributes: plaques, tangles and holes. Based on Dr. Alzheimer's work, key biomarkers of the disease were identified: amyloid beta that forms the amyloid plaques (Chapter 6) and tau which forms the tangles (Chapter 7). Through careful research coupled with serendipity, new biomarkers may also be revealed.

The Search for Causes and Predictors

A key goal in Alzheimer's research is to find consistent and accurate biomarkers that can predict the onset and rate of progress of the disease. One of the problems that biomedical researchers must face is when one gene is mutated or otherwise changed it can affect other genes. The same goes for proteins encoded by these genes. A change in one protein will almost always affect any other proteins or molecules that are regulated by it or which bind to it. This is the so-called pleiotropic effect. To make an analogy, when you remove the battery in your car or when it lacks a charge, many things are affected. The car won't start. The lights don't work; neither does the radio. So one significant change can affect many other things, making it difficult to determine which change actually started the problem. With a simple mechanical device it is easy to work backwards to solve the problem. This isn't the case with people. So the search is on for the triggering event that initiates the onset of Alzheimer's disease. Hopefully a single protein or other individual molecule will be identified as the culprit that starts the downward path to mild cognitive impairment and dementia. However, it is more likely that there are many different routes to Alzheimer's disease and many different triggers that can start the disease process.

Presently, and as we've mentioned in previous chapters, there are only a few different molecules and technologies that have shown potential value as biomarkers. Clearly, different biomarkers appear at different times and each undergoes different patterns of expression. The Alzheimer's disease-related changes in a few of these are summarized in the following figure (Figure 11.3).

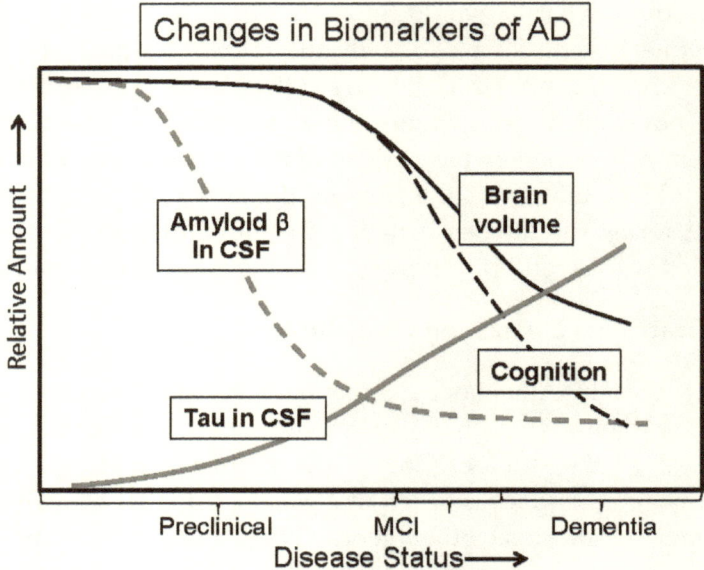

Figure 11.3. Changes in biomarkers at different stages of Alzheimer's disease. CSF, cerebrospinal fluid.

Certain biomarkers, like amyloid beta in cerebrospinal fluid (CSF), can be detected in normal or "presymptomatic" individuals who are at the preclinical stage of the disease. As the disease progresses and mild cognitive impairment (MCI) develops, the levels of amyloid beta decrease in the cerebrospinal fluid. In contrast, tau levels increase in the cerebrospinal fluid. These two changes in the cerebrospinal fluid—loss of amyloid beta and increase in tau —are strong indicators of the presence of Alzheimer's. Other individuals show significant changes during mild cognitive impairment such as MRI images that reveal brain shrinkage. Ultimately these changes are reflected in one's decreasing cognitive and functional abilities as revealed by different cognitive and psychological testing methods.

As useful as these approaches are, more needs to be learned so that these biomarkers can be made more meaningful. It is also possible that new biomarkers can be developed which give more insight into the start and progression of the disease. So just what are the issues faced by researchers in their quest to find appropriate biomarkers?

Required Attributes of Biomarkers

A biomarker needs to meet several criteria to be useful. The biomarker has to be validated as a meaningful predictor of disease onset or as an accurate diagnostic to measure its progression. The biomarker has to serve as a highly reproducible and accurate predictor or diagnostic. It also has to result in low levels of false positives. It can be just as devastating to a person to be told they have a major disease when they don't as it is to be told they actually have that disease. Many tragic events have followed from incorrect information given to patients or relied upon by doctors. So accuracy, without any issue of confusion, is critical.

Once a biomarker has been defined then to ensure this accuracy, the methods for measuring, assessing or detecting that biomarker need to be optimized. The more sensitive the detection method, the better predictor the biomarker becomes. In addition, standardized methods for detecting that biomarker need to be developed that can be applied universally. This is extremely important for research into the causes and cures of any disease. It is also critical in current research as the search for the best biomarker of Alzheimer's disease continues. Dozens of research teams and thousands of researchers worldwide adhere to these goals and are applying them in international studies. While most of the ongoing studies currently use the aforementioned, established biomarkers (Figure 11.1), others are using this approach in the hopes of defining the biomarkers of the future.

Biochemical Biomarkers: Assessing Preclinical Stages

How do you detect if a disease will occur if you don't know what causes the disease? Various academic consortia worldwide are working on this problem. As we've discussed, a prime suspect for a causal agent in Alzheimer's disease is the accumulation of amyloid beta (A3). More specifically, the 42-amino-acid version or $A\beta42$ is of primary interest. To refresh your memory, this peptide is produced then it clumps into amyloid plaques which can induce specific changes in nerve cells leading to their malfunction and death. This inability to function and death of neurons underlies the brain changes that are reflected as cognitive impairment.

So using amyloid beta as our biomarker, let's look at some of the ways its progression to plaque formation and impact on the Alzheimer's sufferer can be followed (Figure 11.4).

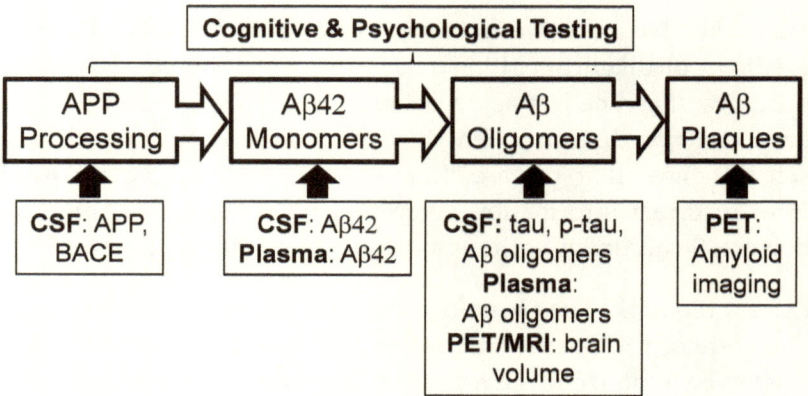

Figure 11.4. Tracking amyloid beta cascade biomarkers as indicators of Alzheimer's disease. Aβ, amyloid beta; APP, amyloid protein precursor; CSF, cerebrospinal fluid; BACE, beta-secretase; MRI, magnetic resonance imaging; PET, positron emission tomography. (Modified from Cummings et al., 2011)

Thus the appearance or increase in Aβ42 in the brain is considered a hallmark of the onset of Alzheimer's disease. For this reason the peptide Aβ42 is a major biomarker for the disease. A decrease in this biomarker peptide in cerebrospinal fluid or its detection via PET imaging in the brain can be taken as evidence that future cognitive impairment leading to Alzheimer's disease is a distinct possibility.

Tracking the Movements of Amyloid Beta

As noted in the previous section, various biomarkers in the amyloid cascade leading to plaque formation can be used. While the final area of concern is the accumulation of amyloid beta monomers, oligomers and plaques in the brain, the biomarkers used don't always involve brain tissue. In fact for the earliest biomarker detection, cerebrospinal fluid and plasma levels of amyloid protein precursor (APP), beta-secretase (BACE) and Aβ42 are estimated. This is because these molecules are found in many tissues in the body, not just the brain. As a result the improper processing of amyloid precursor protein and the involvement of beta-secretase can lead to Aβ42 formation in those tissues. As with many such molecules, amyloid beta peptides can leave those tissues and enter the bloodstream. They can also move from the bloodstream into the cerebrospinal fluid and the brain. These transfers of amyloid beta between various bodily compartments are summarized in Figure 11.5.

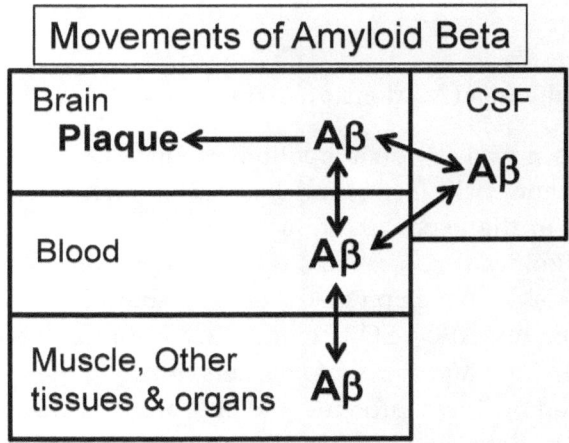

Figure 11.5. Amyloid beta is produced in a diversity of human tissues and can move between them to accumulate in the brain as a natural event or as a precursor to the formation of plaque. (Modified from Cummings et al., 2011)

A great deal is known about the way amyloid beta is processed in these different compartments and how it moves between them. For us, what is important about this information is that the movements between these compartments become altered in Alzheimer's disease. As an example, in normal individuals the amyloid beta content of the cerebrospinal fluid is completely turned over (replaced) about two times every day. In the normal brain it is broken down by a diversity of enzymes as well as lost through transfer to other compartments. Most of the blood amyloid beta comes from the brain but a small amount comes from cerebrospinal fluid as well as various tissues and organs.

In Alzheimer's many changes occur that affect the turnover of amyloid beta, but of concern here is that when Aβ42 is formed it doesn't get broken down or turned over as efficiently. As a result it primarily gets incorporated into amyloid plaques. The result of this is that Aβ42 levels in the cerebrospinal fluid drop because the peptide is now trapped in brain plaques and unavailable to move into this bodily compartment. So a drop in cerebrospinal fluid amyloid beta is one important biomarker for Alzheimer's. On the other hand, serum levels of Aβ42 do not seem to undergo significant changes, making this a poor indicator for the progression of MCI to dementia.

Other Biochemical Markers of Alzheimer's

The presence of the protein apolipoprotein E (APOE) is another major genetic risk factor for late-onset Alzheimer's disease. Mutations in the genes encoding presenilin-1 and -2 (PSN-1/-2) are also significant risk factors. (Other biomarkers indicating an increased risk of developing Alzheimer's comprise an additional list of acronyms: APOJ, SORL1, and PICALM.) As a result, APOE and PSN-1/-2 are additional biomarkers linked to the disease. The genes encoding these proteins and the proteins themselves are discussed in detail in Chapter 13. As biomarkers of the disease, we would expect to see increases in their levels to coincide with an increase in cognitive decline. How do we assess their presence and/or increase in their levels? For the most part the answer to this question is not yet available.

Brain Imaging as a Biomarker

Alzheimer's disease involves more than just impairment of cognitive function. It also involves changes in brain-controlled physiological events in the body such as altered patterns of sleep as well as increases in epilepsy and seizure activity. Fundamentally, all of these changes reflect altered brain function that can be evaluated using various neuroimaging techniques. In fact it is currently argued by some that neuroimaging is the best way to assess the progression of Alzheimer's. These issues are the focus of the Alzheimer's disease neuroimaging initiative (www.adni-info.org), a selfless conglomeration of scientists whose goal is to share information. Unlike for-profit organizations, these scientists freely share what they learn and forgo any rights to their discoveries. Information gained from the analysis and validation of data collected by MRI and PET imaging as well as results from assessments of biomarkers in the blood and cerebrospinal fluid are available on their website.

Neuroimaging may also be the best way, at present, to determine the earliest stages of onset of the disease. As mentioned, the onset was believed to occur as many as ten years prior to the appearance of any symptoms of the disease but may in fact begin decades before any symptoms are evident. At present there are a group of neuroimaging methods that dominate the Alzheimer's disease landscape along with a number of others that are being developed. Our goal is to make the reader aware of how these techniques work at a basic level and how they are being used in the evaluation of Alzheimer's disease. We'll also see some of the hope that's on the horizon.

There are three main types of brain imaging that are used to evaluate the presence or absence of Alzheimer's disease. They are also used in evaluating the success of clinical trials and in studying the progress of the disease. The three are Magnetic Resonance Imaging (MRI), Positron Emission Tomography (PET) and Electroencephalogram (EEG). We'll look at each of them in terms of their value as a method for evaluating the existence of Alzheimer's as well as assessing early events that might lead to the disease.

Magnetic Resonance Imaging (MRI)

Magnetic resonance imaging (MRI) is a relatively non-invasive technique that is used to visualize internal body structures. It is particularly useful in studying the brain and so has become a valuable tool in studying and assessing the status of the Alzheimer's brain. MRI scanners are devices that use large and powerful magnets. Without getting too technical, they align the positively-charged protons in bodily molecules. Of these, water is the primary proton-containing molecule that is affected. When the MRI scanner is turned on, the magnets align the water molecules. When the magnet is turned off, the molecules return back to their unaligned state. During this relaxation phase a radio frequency signal is sent out that can be measured. Computer programs using high-level mathematics allow the results to be converted into understandable images. The placement of the magnets can be altered to generate 3D images of the brain. This is used, for example, to detect relatively small regions of the brain in detail. Since MRI does not employ ionizing radiation, as do X-rays and CT scans, it is considered to be a relatively safe procedure. Purchasing and setting up an MRI facility is not cheap, with a single machine and suite costing somewhere around two to three million dollars or more.

There are many types of MRI approaches that are available but fundamentally they can be grouped into two classes: structural (sMRI) and functional (fMRI). As the name implies, structural approaches reveal aspects of brain structure including overall size and the sizes of various specific regions and ventricles, for example (See Figures 4.3, 4.4 in Chapter 4). Thus MRI can assess brain atrophy but the overall decrease in the amount of brain tissue is not by itself an indicator of Alzheimer's disease. Brain volume decreases in all of us as we age. In contrast, atrophy of the hippocampus does indicate the presence of Alzheimer's disease; atrophy of the hippocampus also occurs more rapidly with Alzheimer's dementia than it does in healthy individuals of the same relative age. Ventricular volume also increases as we age. The rate of ventricular enlargement however is about two times faster in Alzheimer's individuals whose main symptom is memory loss, a type referred to as amnesic MCI. More significantly, the rate of ventricular enlargement is over six times greater in those who suffer from Alzheimer's dementia. As detailed in Chapter 4, Alzheimer's disease is also associated with the thinning of the cortex of the brain, another structural change that can be assessed by certain types of MRI. Follow-up autopsy data reveal that the brain changes linked to the progression of Alzheimer's disease as assessed by MRI and verified by cognitive testing correlate well with the amount of neurofibrillary tangles but, for some reason, not with amyloid plaque levels.

The second area where MRI is valuable is in assessing brain function. As opposed to simply looking at brain structure, functional MRI "sees" brain cells in action. It is a way of visualizing the changing neural activity of the brain. The common way this is done is via a method called task-activated BOLD (Blood Oxygen Level-Dependent) signaling. When a brain region is active, oxygenated blood flows there and this is detected as a positive signal on a functional MRI scan. Thus, whatever we do using our brains—talk, think, decide, answer questions, etc.—specific brain regions light up in functional MRI scans because of blood flowing into them. Where structural MRI is a valuable tool for assessing the structural changes in the brain during MCI and the transition to dementia, functional MRI holds the promise of defining the earliest changes in the brain that are a prelude to the clinical manifestations of the disease.

Episodic versus Semantic Memory

Studies on functional MRI have historically relied on the assessment of an individual's brain changes in response to testing or completing tasks involving either episodic memory or semantic memory. Episodic memory involves the ability to distinguish between previously learned information as opposed to new material. In other words, if we think of our lives like a story made up of many individual episodes, it involves the memory of things we have experienced throughout our lives. Impairment in episodic memory is another hallmark of Alzheimer's disease and thus a decline in episodic memory can be indicative of existing mild cognitive impairment. However, issues occur with the testing paradigm for various reasons, one of which is simply that individuals who are being tested often find that the challenge of responding causes them to mentally "freeze up", skewing the results of the data. This is because declines in episodic memory are also common in the normal aging process.

Semantic memory reflects our knowledge about and understanding of the world around us. Our life experiences have allowed us to develop concepts that can be applied to things even though we might never have experienced them. Thus functional MRI testing might involve discriminating between real words and made-up words or between the faces of famous people versus unknown individuals. Unlike episodic memory, semantic memory remains relatively intact as we age but is usually affected in Alzheimer's individuals. Thus functional MRI holds out hope for detecting the earliest events in loss of cognition before there has been any clinical manifestation of the disease.

Functional versus Structural MRI

Since functional MRI requires more extensive expertise and relies more heavily on patient cooperation than structural MRI, it has only been useful for small studies. There are many reasons that functional MRI has its detractors. Because many different regions light up as blobs of color in brain images, some less-than-kind neuroscientists refer to functional MRI as "Blobology". One of the other concerns brought to light for functional MRI studies is the experimental design and how it is applied. Many studies have generated what at first glance appear to be contradictory findings. One reason for this is that experimenters often used different types of evaluators (e.g., naming items versus face recognition) and/or failed to take into consideration the type and extent of the brain or cognitive changes that have occurred in each individual in the test cohort. In other words, they attempted to draw the same conclusions while studying different things. In addition, the boost in blood flow to various brain regions is often difficult to separate from background noise which can also be a reason different researchers get different results or, at least, interpret them differently. A valuable early biomarker needs to be based on accurate and unquestionable interpretation. On the other hand, this is what early studies often do—they reveal what needs to be controlled for and considered in carrying out future experiments.

In summary, structural MRI is valuable in assessing structural changes in the brain that occur in MCI and how these changes progress. In contrast, functional MRI looks at functional aspects of the brain and, while the technique is still developing and has its detractors, hopefully one day it will guide researchers to finding biomarkers of the earliest phases of Alzheimer's disease onset. Thus MRI, whether structural or functional, serves not only as a valuable method in the assessment of the disease but also in the interpretation of results from clinical trials.

PET Scans

Positron emission tomography or PET has a number of biomedical uses, but in the detection or study of Alzheimer's disease it is primarily used to detect the presence of amyloid plaques in the brain. PET imaging of brain changes in Alzheimer's disease is based on detecting the localization of radioactively labeled (radiolabeled) compounds that bind to amyloid plaques. As we all know, the use of radioactivity is always a concern. Historically, "Pittsburgh compound B" labeled with radioactive carbon ($[^{11}C]$ PIB) was one of the first agents that used to detect amyloid plaques via PET imaging. A number of variants and other radioactive compounds have been developed and more are under development. Pittsburgh compound B localization is significantly increased in the frontal cortex and other appropriate brain regions of Alzheimer's individuals compared to those who have no symptoms of the disease. Just as important, the compound does not localize to areas that are normally not affected in those with Alzheimer's disease.

Amyloid plaque formation is a relatively early event in the development of Alzheimer's and PET is an excellent way to detect its presence and localization. However, this imaging technique is not useful in following the progression of the disease because once plaques appear they essentially resolve at the maximum detectable level for PET imaging, so assessing further increases or changes is not possible. There are other issues as well. Many elderly people who are cognitively normal, showing no evidence of neurodegeneration, also have amyloid plaques in their brains. The reason for this is still an issue that is under study.

Sugar for Your PET

The use of radioactively labeled glucose analog (fluorodeoxyglucose or FDG) is also coupled with PET and referred to cleverly as an FDG PET scan. This technique is more commonly used to detect and study cancers since the uptake of glucose is greatest in these actively dividing cells. Glucose also is taken up in active areas of the brain. With Alzheimer's disease, specific regions of the brain will show reduced levels of sugar uptake as summarized in Figure 11.6. Typically, active areas show up as red with less active areas tending towards orange and green. Brain ventricles show up as blue to black areas. Thus, FDG PET images reveal how much loss of neuronal activity has occurred in specific regions of the Alzheimer's brain.

Normal Aging vs. Alzheimer's Disease
FDG PET Scan of Brain

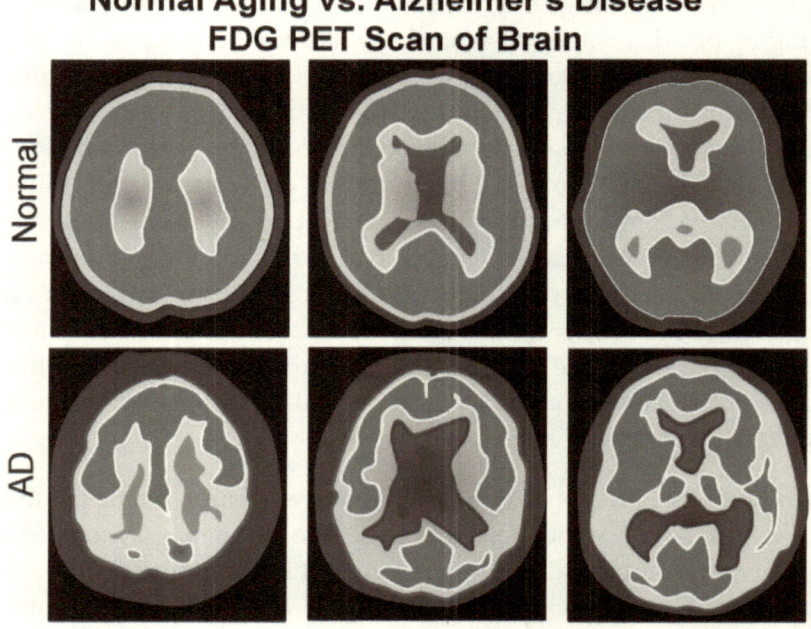

Figure 11.6. Diagram of FDG PET scans of Alzheimer's versus normal brains. FDG, fluorodeoxyglucose; PET, positron emission tomography. (After Peterson, R.C., 2011)

Typically, detection is via PET scan but also single-photon emission tomography or SPECT can and is used. That said, PET is used more commonly because it provides greater sensitivity and resolution. In addition, more tracers have been and are being developed for PET as compared to SPECT. One future goal of tracer development is to find compounds that bind to different plaque attributes or other proteins that are present in plaques. (These other proteins were discussed in Chapter 6). Using two tracers also could be employed in PET scans to provide more insight into plaque formation and its progression in those with Alzheimer's.

The big problem facing the development of new PET tracers is making compounds that can cross the blood–brain barrier. As its name implies, this is a barrier that prevents molecules and cells from leaving the blood and entering the brain. On the other hand it does allow small, specific, usually hydrophobic molecules like oxygen, carbon dioxide and specific hormones to cross. Dyes such as thioflavin T, Congo red and chrysamine G are all small hydrophobic molecules that can cross the blood–brain barrier. Historically, each of these dyes has been used in histological sections to detect amyloid plaques in brain tissue after autopsy. To detect plaques in living tissues, radioactive label has to be added so that these dyes can be detected via PET scan.

EEG: Electrical Imaging of the Alzheimer's Brain

Brain function can be assessed by its electrical activity, so the use of electroencephalography (EEG) has become a useful tool not only in evaluating the clinical progression of the disease. EEG is also being used for the detection of electrical changes that can serve as Alzheimer's disease biomarkers. Of course, this all started with the work of the famous physician and physicist Luigi Galvani who learned that the muscles of dead frogs could contract ("twitch") when stimulated with electricity. Not to wander off topic, but Galvani's pure research set the stage for EEG development and all the wondrous advances it has spawned in both medicine and biomedical research. It is the primary reason why pure research needs to be funded at a high level—because the majority of advances in science have come from such basic work which set the stage for future useful applications. So Galvani set the stage but it took the German, Hans Berger, to transform the concept of electrical flow in nerve cells to develop the first EEG ("Elektrenkephalogramm").

EEG is a non-invasive way to measure brain patterns and activity. Electrodes connected to recorders are placed on the scalp and the electrical activity of the brain under various conditions is then measured. There are daily (circadian) patterns of brain activity that are well defined for both normal and various medical conditions. Humans also display specific patterns of activity during sleep so it's possible to designate the progression (stages) of sleep as well as its depth. So stage one is the earliest stage and stage four is the deepest stage of sleep. Rapid eye movement (REM) associated with dreaming is also evident as specific patterns on an EEG. Since sleep patterns are altered with Alzheimer's disease, these changes can be detected using an electroencephalogram. When the brain is active during certain behaviors, other patterns of electrical activity appear that are appropriate to that behavior. The Alzheimer's brain shows altered patterns during such behaviors. Similarly, various medical, physiological and behavioral conditions are also reflected in patterns that stray from the norm. For example, as noted above, the progression of Alzheimer's is linked to increases in epilepsy and seizures. In keeping with this, those suffering from the disease show increases in epileptiform and seizure patterns in EEGs.

Today, quantitative electroencephalography (qEEG) has upped the ante in the development of diagnostic evaluation of clinical Alzheimer's. It also offers clues to finding specific biomarkers for the early stages of MCI. For example, in relation to altered sleep patterns, quantitative electroencephalography can reveal the loss of stage two sleep features linked to Alzheimer's. These patterns are distinct to the disease and not simply to aging. The quantitative electroencephalography changes that have been detected in Alzheimer's brain patterns are strongly correlated with other biomarkers, especially the levels of tau and phosphorylated tau protein in cerebrospinal fluid. So it is possible that quantitative electroencephalography biomarkers could also be combined with other types of biomarkers to determine the earliest brain changes that are related to the onset of the disease. REM sleep is also altered in Alzheimer's individuals. More normal dreaming can be restored with specific pharmaceuticals such as acetylcholinesterase inhibitors (e.g., donepezil) and NMDA antagonists (e.g., memantine) and this is reflected in restored REM patterns as measured by EEGs.

There is increasing evidence that quantitative electroencephalography measures of brain activity in the cortex may be used not only to distinguish Alzheimer's individuals from normal, healthy individuals but also to classify Alzheimer's patients as to the stage of development of the disease. From such work a simple, non-invasive quantitative electroencephalography biomarker may be developed that can be coupled with a non-invasive biochemical biomarker (e.g., a protein/peptide change in saliva?) to predict the earliest stages of Alzheimer's disease.

Cognitive Self-Testing for Alzheimer's Disease

Early identification of memory impairment and other cognitive problems is another way to assess the potential development of Alzheimer's as well as other neurological diseases. Tests which assess one's ability to process information can give insight into a person's cognitive status. Similarly, assessing one's memory, the ability to reason and the ability to switch from one task to another can tell whether one's cognitive ability is normal or not. Obviously having such tests done early in life to be followed up in later years would be more useful than a single test but, regardless, valuable insight can be gained either way.

As we age, we all worry about our level of forgetfulness. Is it a sign of some serious underlying change such as the onset of Alzheimer's or is it just part of getting older? When a person has any concerns about their cognitive ability they should talk with their doctor. If this is not possible or not desirable, then one can use self-testing as a way to either ease one's mind or reinforce the need for an expert opinion. Many Alzheimer societies have cognitive self-tests available on their websites. For example, www.alz.org has three preliminary cognitive tests on its website that are designed for use by doctors but can be used by individuals together with a family member or friend. The tests are quick and simple. They include a three-word delayed recall exercise where you are given three common nouns and asked to recall them after five minutes. A variant of this, called the "mini-cog", involves drawing the face of a clock with a given time before being asked to recall the three words. The third is a coin-counting exercise where you are asked to total a series of coins in random order (i.e., not ascending or descending order of value). These simple tests evaluate comprehension, working memory, recall, planning and calculating skills. If you have any concerns after evaluating your responses to the online testing, you would be wise to confer with your doctor for guidance.

Formal Cognitive Screening

It is important to realize that cognitive testing can reveal if there is any significant decline in one's ability to remember, calculate or comprehend. On their own, such tests cannot establish whether this decline is due to Alzheimer's disease or some other problem. Determining why there is a change in one's cognitive ability requires testing for other biomarkers as detailed above. However, cognitive testing plays a critical part in establishing whether the disease is underway or not.

The following summarizes some of the many formal cognitive tests that exist:

1. **MMSE**: Mini-Mental State Examination. This short test (~10 min.) evaluates various aspects of cognition including attention, calculation, language abilities, visual construction and word recall.

2. **MoCA**: Montreal Cognitive Assessment. Another relatively simple and short test, MoCA can help medical professionals assess whether a person suffers from abnormal cognitive function. It can predict dementia in individuals with MCI.

3. **SLUMS**: Saint Louis University Mental Status Exam. This 11-item test includes items such as recognition of geometric figures and naming animals, among other things. It is valuable in assessing individuals with MCI.

4. **ADAS-Cog**: Alzheimer's Disease Assessment Scale—Cognitive Test. Consisting of 11 parts and being more thorough than the MMSE, this test takes about half an hour and can reveal individuals with MCI. It is a strong test for memory and language skills.

When there is concern about a person's cognitive ability, a variety of tests may be employed that are administered by a psychologist who specializes in cognitive disorders (neuropsychologist). These can precisely define aspects of the problem and direct the physician to proper care for their patient.

The Biomarker Future

The best biomarker for any disease is something that accurately detects the disease and can be measured precisely in a freely available bodily fluid like saliva or blood. For Alzheimer's disease, the identification of a molecule that triggers the disease or appears very early during its onset would be the best bet. To date, no such molecule exists and it is not likely a single molecular indicator will ever be found. At present, neuroimaging is the best indicator of changes in the brain that signal the future onset of Alzheimer's. However, this is a relatively expensive, time-consuming procedure that can't be used as a one-off diagnosis. With the development of new, rapid and definitive neuroimaging approaches, these problems will likely be diminished. In contrast, while current biomarker approaches focusing on amyloid beta and its gang members are allowing biomedical researchers and MDs to define the existence of Alzheimer's, they currently are providing information that is too late to set the stage for preventing disease onset, let alone a cure. Recent work suggests we may have to start our search for a cause much earlier than previously thought.

Alzheimer's May Start Decades before Any Symptoms

To date, the biomedical message has been that the cause(s) of Alzheimer's disease appears a decade or so before any symptoms are detectable. That presumption was turned on its head in the fall of 2012 with the publishing of a paper that showed that some Alzheimer's biomarkers begin to appear decades prior to the appearance of symptoms. The study involved a group of 18- to 26-year-olds at genetic risk for early-onset Alzheimer's disease and an equivalent control group that lacked the mutated presenilin-1 gene (PSEN1, see Chapter 12). Both groups were free of any cognitive impairment. Those who were genetically at risk showed high levels of fibrillar amyloid beta in appropriate brain regions while this harmful peptide was absent from the brains of the control group. These results indicate that amyloid beta accumulation in the brain can begin decades prior to any signs or symptoms.

This study provides hope for those at genetic risk for early onset because the window of opportunity for dealing with the disease now is evidently much greater than previously realized. Of course, this information is of limited use until an effective drug for slowing or stopping the progress of the disease is available. Some consider the results as being translatable to understanding late-onset Alzheimer's disease, which accounts for 95% of individuals who get the disease. However, this may not be reasonable since the study involved early-onset subjects and there are significant differences between early- and late-onset Alzheimer's. Still, this new insight, as with any research that advances our understanding of the disease, can only help as researchers continue in their search for the elusive non-genetic driving forces behind Alzheimer's disease. Until that is successful, biomarkers can help us diagnose the disease; but without a cure, the diagnosis remains of limited value.

Chapter 12

Searching for Alzheimer's Genes

The primary focus of Alzheimer's disease research internationally is on the formation of amyloid plaques and neurofibrillary tangles in the brain—these are the central recognized culprits of the disease. Amyloid plaques are the predominant structures that form between brain cells in Alzheimer's sufferers. Neurofibrillary tangles are the major components that form within their brain cells. Most believe that plaque formation precedes tangle production. As scientists began to probe into the ways these plaques and tangles form in the Alzheimer's brain, it became clear that they are not simple biochemical processes. (The basic steps in plaque [Chapter 6] and tangle [Chapter 7] formation were covered earlier in the book.) As we move ahead and each step is revealed, new avenues are opened and new regulatory targets are exposed. Which pathways should scientists follow? At present no one can answer that question. So here we will look first at the kinds of genetic research that are being done and the promises they hold.

Genetic Links to Alzheimer's Disease

It is interesting that the earliest isolation of amyloid beta was done using the brain from a trisomy 21 (Down syndrome) person. The first isolation of the peptide from the brain of a person with a late-onset Alzheimer's disease was done by the same group using meningeal blood vessels. These initial identifications linking amyloid beta to Alzheimer's disease were done in 1984, setting the stage for work that is ongoing today. The history behind this original research and the evolution of the understanding of the genetics of Alzheimer's disease gives novel insight into how biomedical research progresses with starts and stops and, even, erroneous initial viewpoints.

* * *

FYI: Naming Genes versus Proteins

Generally the names of genes are italicized as shown in Table 12.1 while the protein name is not. Since this is not a scientific publication, for simplicity italics are not used for gene names. Instead, if it is important to note that we are talking about a gene, then this will be clarified (e.g., "a gene encoding" or "the gene for", etc.).

* * *

There is an inherited component to both early- and late-onset Alzheimer's disease. It is believed that between 65–79% of cases are caused by genetic mutations. In spite of this there is no clear understanding of how genetics define the disease, especially for late-onset Alzheimer's. This is likely due to the fact the disease is heterogeneous and very complex. So complex that some consider it a syndrome rather than a disease. While the overwhelming majority of cases of the disease are late onset, there is little direct evidence for a clearly defined heritable component. This is because there likely is a large number of susceptibility genes involved rather than one or two causative genes. In spite of this, a few genes have consistently been shown to increase the risk of getting the late-onset form of the disease. The risk genes linked to late-onset Alzheimer's disease are listed in Table 12.1. Of these, a gene encoding a variant of a protein called apolipoprotein E (APOE; also commonly written as ApoE) demonstrates the tightest relationship with the development of the late-onset form of the disease. Acetylcholinesterase which is central to nerve function is also linked to Alzheimer's and is a major target in pharmacotherapy (Chapter 9). Other genes linked to Alzheimer's disease are also of central interest and are detailed below.

Genetic Links to Alzheimer's Disease

Early-Onset AD

Protein (*gene*)	Function
Amyloid protein precursor (*APP*)	Source of amyloid beta
Presenilin-1 (*PSEN1*)	Subunit of γ-secretase
Presenilin-2 (*PSEN2*)	Subunit of γ-secretase

Down Syndrome AD

Protein (*gene*)	Function
Amyloid protein precursor (*APP*)	Source of amyloid beta
Calcineurin A (*CNA*)	Dephosphorylates tau, other proteins
Apolipoprotein E (*ApoE*)	Lipid/cholesterol metabolism

Late-Onset AD

Protein (*gene*)	Function
Apolipoprotein E (*ApoE*))	Lipid/cholesterol metabolism
Acetylcholinesterase	Breakdown of acetylcholine
SORL1	amyloid beta uptake by cells
Others (*ABCA7, BIN1, CD33, CD2AP, CLU, CR1, EPHA1, MS4A4E/MS4A6A* and *PICALM*)	Various functions: see text

---

Table 12.1. The primary genes linked to early-onset and late-onset and Down syndrome Alzheimer's disease.

In contrast, with early-onset Alzheimer's disease, which typically occurs before the age of 65, there is undisputed evidence for a direct role of inheritance. In scientific terms this is called Mendelian inheritance. It is where normal and abnormal genes are directly passed down to children from their parents. For early-onset Alzheimer's disease, there are three main genetic culprits that make people at risk and they are all involved in the production of amyloid beta, the precursor of amyloid plaques. These are listed in Table 12.1. Mutations in the gene for amyloid precursor protein or APP are one link to early-onset Alzheimer's disease. As detailed in Chapter 6, amyloid precursor protein is the precursor to amyloid beta. As a result, any mutations that affect the processing of amyloid precursor protein can affect the level of production of the harmful peptide. The other two mutations that are of particular interest occur in genes encoding the proteins presenilin-1 (PSEN1) and -2 (PSEN2). As detailed below, these presenilins are the enzymatic part of gamma-secretase, the final enzyme in the sequence that cleaves amyloid precursor protein to release amyloid beta peptides.

A type of early-onset Alzheimer's disease is also intimately associated with Down syndrome. In addition to the genes for amyloid precursor protein and apolipoprotein E, the gene encoding an enzyme called calcineurin is tightly associated with Down syndrome Alzheimer's disease (Table 12.1). These genes are detailed in the following sections.

In spite of some basic similarities between late-onset, early-onset and Down syndrome Alzheimer's, it is widely believed that they are fundamentally different. In spite of this the overlap of specific genes (APOE, late-onset and Down syndrome Alzheimer's disease; amyloid precursor protein, early-onset and Down syndrome Alzheimer's disease) suggests there may be some similarities worth studying. There is a genetic link between neurofibrillary tangle formation and Down syndrome Alzheimer's disease. In contrast, it is interesting to note, no candidate genes for tangle formation have been universally linked to early-onset or late-onset forms of the disease. Now let's begin with an examination of Down syndrome Alzheimer's disease, after which early-onset and late-onset Alzheimer's disease will be detailed.

Down Syndrome and Alzheimer's Disease

If there ever was evidence for a genetic link for Alzheimer's disease, it was provided by Down syndrome. The relationship between Down syndrome (DS) and Alzheimer's disease has been well established and early-onset Alzheimer's disease is common in those with this genetic condition. In keeping with the major markers of Alzheimer's, the brains of Down syndrome individuals who are suffering from the disease possess amyloid plaques and neurofibrillary tangles. Based on this and other attributes, some have suggested that Down syndrome can serve as a model for understanding at least some of the aspects of the start and progress of Alzheimer's disease. So before looking at this in detail, a short introduction to Down syndrome is in order.

Down syndrome is referred to medically as trisomy 21. Thus, as its alternative name indicates, Down syndrome is due to an extra copy of chromosome 21. It is a result of the improper separation of chromosomes, called non-disjunction. Most cases of non-disjunction are due to the "maternal age effect". Older women have higher incidences of abnormal chromosome numbers in their eggs due to those eggs being held in a suspended state (i.e., meiosis II) for an extended period of time. In 95% of cases, Down syndrome is caused by the meiotic non-disjunction during egg maturation in the ovaries. This means that during normal cell division, certain chromosomes don't pull apart properly. This results in erroneous sorting of the chromosomes leading to abnormal numbers of chromosomes in the offspring cells. As a result, typically one cell gets two chromosomes while the other cell doesn't get that chromosome. For example, when the resultant egg has an extra chromosome (i.e., 24 rather than the normal 23) and it is fertilized, the male sperm will contribute another copy of that chromosome. This results in three copies of the same chromosome. The resulting syndrome is called trisomy ("tri" or three; "somy", chromosomes).

So people with Down syndrome have three copies of chromosome 21. There are 225 genes on this chromosome. The extra copy of each one of these genes affects development of brain, immune system, heart and skeleton. One of the genes on chromosome 21 that is involved in some of these effects was give the name "Down Syndrome Critical Region 1" or DSCR1. One function of DSCR1 is in the development of brain nerve cells. The extra copy of DSCR1 leads to the overproduction of DSCR1 protein in developing brain cells which leads to abnormal neuron development—the underlying cause of the cognitive problems faced by Down syndrome individuals.

The Link to Tangle Formation

There's more to the DSCR1 story. DSCR1 may trigger some of the neurodegenerative events associated with Alzheimer's disease. A diversity of lines of research has implicated calcineurin as a critical enzyme that dephosphorylates tau. As a result, this enzyme is believed to function in preventing neurofibrillary tangles. In Down syndrome, excess DSCR1 causes the inhibition of calcineurin. Its inhibition would prevent calcineurin from removing phosphate groups from tau which in turn would allow neurofibrillary tangle formation to proceed unchecked.

But DSCR1 isn't the only gene that affects normal brain development. There is a genetic link between Down syndrome, the amyloid precursor protein and apolipoprotein E genes as well. A gene for amyloid protein precursor is also encoded on chromosome 21. As a result, this protein that serves as a precursor to the formation of soluble amyloid beta, which is the essence of plaque formation, is over-expressed. As a result most people with Down syndrome have high levels of amyloid beta by the time they are 30 years old. In some cases diffuse amyloid plaques are seen in Down syndrome children as young as twelve.

There are between five and eight million people with Down syndrome worldwide. Since individuals with Down syndrome are living longer these days, the incidence of neurodegenerative diseases is increasing within this group. Because this group expresses many different symptoms, particular attention will have to be made by society to address their needs. Currently there are very few drug studies done with them as a focus group. This is important to consider because due to their neuropathological attributes, they may respond differently to different pharmaceuticals than others.

Three Bad Genes Linked to Early-Onset Alzheimer's

The first genes that were identified as being linked to Alzheimer's disease are APP, PSEN1 and PSEN2. Mutations in any one of these three genes can lead to what is termed autosomal dominant Alzheimer's disease. This is an early-onset genetically linked (or familial form) of the disease. That said, the accumulated data indicate that mutations in APP and the presenilins are responsible for only a small proportion of early-onset Alzheimer's disease. Each of these three proteins is intimately associated with the formation of amyloid beta, the nasty little peptide that is the basis of amyloid plaques that form in the Alzheimer's brain. The APP gene encodes amyloid precursor protein, the protein from which amyloid beta is extracted as a prelude to amyloid plaque formation.

At this time, two dozen mutations in the APP gene have been shown to cause Alzheimer's disease. It is interesting that most of the APP mutations are clustered in a small region of the protein in or around the amyloid beta site.

While we have been talking about amyloid beta in general terms, as covered in Chapter 6, in reality there are two main amyloid beta troublemakers: Aβ42 and Aβ40. The 42 and 40 refer to amyloid peptides of 42 and 40 amino acids in length, respectively. Aβ42 is the bigger troublemaker. As you might expect, certain APP mutations result in the formation of excess Aβ42 as a prelude to plaque formation. Other mutations cause the resulting amyloid beta peptides that are formed to be stickier causing them to aggregate more quickly and, as a result, for plaques to form more easily. There are autopsy data revealing greater amounts of amyloid in people with early-onset Alzheimer's disease caused by APP mutations compared to those who had the late-onset or sporadic form of the disease. While APP mutations are a cause of early-onset familial Alzheimer's disease, these mutations account for only a minority of autosomal dominant forms of the disease. This prompted researchers to look for other culprits.

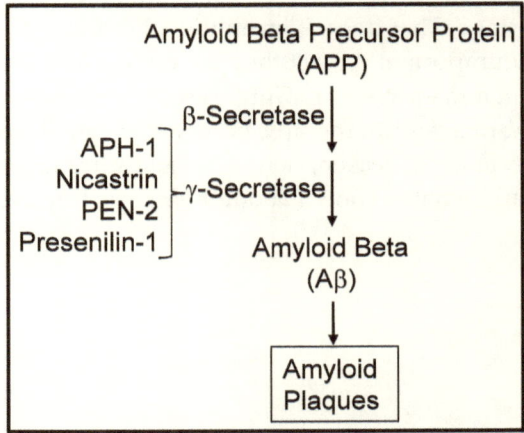

Figure 12.1. The processing of amyloid precursor protein (APP) by beta-secretase and gamma-secretase to release amyloid beta peptides. While beta-secretase is comprised of a single protein, gamma-secretase is a multi-protein enzyme made up of APH-1, nicastrin, PEN-2 and presenilin as detailed in the text.

The processing of APP by gamma-secretase and beta-secretase results in the formation of amyloid beta peptides as detailed in Chapter 6. As shown in Figure 12.1, we can add to that story here. The portion of APP that hangs outside of nerve cells is first chopped off by beta-secretase. Then gamma-secretase cuts off the smaller amyloid beta peptide, releasing it to the extracellular environment as a prelude to amyloid plaque formation. While beta-secretase is an enzyme comprised of a single protein, gamma-secretase is a multi-protein complex. It took many years of research to reveal that gamma-secretase is actually made up of four protein subunits: APH-1 (anterior pharynx defective-1), nicastrin, PEN-2 (presenilin enhancer-2) and presenilin-1. Now we will focus on the presenilins. While they are not germane to our discussion here, the other gamma-secretase proteins are discussed in the following FYI section (FYI: The Other Proteins of Gamma-Secretase).

* * *

FYI: The Other Proteins of Gamma-Secretase

Gamma-secretase is involved in the second and final processing step of APP to produce amyloid beta. Since presenilin mutations have been linked to the early onset of Alzheimer's disease, they have taken center stage. That doesn't mean the other three proteins of this enzyme are unimportant. In fact they are critical to the structure and function of gamma-secretase. Until research reveals their use as targets for pharmaceutical therapy, however, they will continue to be second string. For that reason, here we'll just summarize what these proteins are and what is known about their basic function.

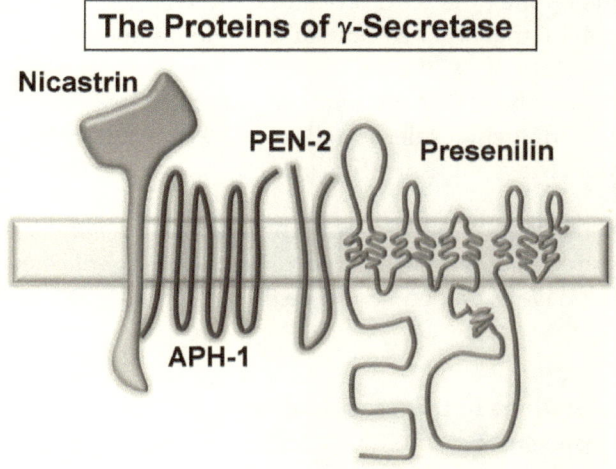

Figure 12.2. The proteins that make up gamma-secretase.
The way these proteins associate to form the functional
enzyme is under study. APH-1, anterior pharynx
defective-1; PEN-2, presenilin enhancer-2.

APH-1 is one of the four proteins that constitute gamma-secretase
(Figure 12.2). APH-1 was first identified in the tiny nematode called
C. elegans. (This tiny worm has done a lot for science, supporting
arguments for using model systems in biomedical research.)
Mutations in the APH-1 gene resulted in defects in the upper regions
of the throat or pharynx. Hence APH-1 is an acronym for anterior
pharynx defective-1, the first mutation resulting in this defect. As
probably is already evident, the APH-1 gene is highly conserved
since it is found in humans as well, where it functions as part of
gamma-secretase. APH-1 is also involved in the localization of
nicastrin to the cell surface.

Nicastrin was named after a village in Italy called Nicastro. This
place was the site where an extended Italian family was shown to
have a high incidence of familial Alzheimer's disease (FAD). The
largest of the gamma-secretase proteins, nicastrin has been called
"the gatekeeper of gamma-secretase". It is so named because it is
involved in recognizing the piece of APP that is left in the cell
membrane after beta-secretase action, allowing the full gamma-
secretase enzyme to cleave off the small and harmful amyloid beta
peptide.

As its name implies, the third protein PEN-2, or presenilin enhancer-2, is involved in the organization of the membrane-bound gamma-secretase. While it is the smallest of the four gamma-secretase subunits, like the other proteins it has many cellular functions related to fundamental roles in cell-to-cell communication and signal transduction. Most published research has focused on those functions.

While this section provides some information into the proteins of gamma-secretase, it doesn't do true justice to the complex and myriad studies that have been done on these three proteins.

* * *

Specific mutations in the genes encoding the proteins presenilin-1 (PSEN1), presenilin-2 (PSEN2) and amyloid precursor protein (APP) lead to susceptibility for the development of early-onset Alzheimer's disease. In other words, people who have certain mutations in those genes have a much greater chance of getting Alzheimer's later in life. However, the types of mutations and the genes affected lead to different ways the disease presents itself and to different resulting pathological features. Evaluating the changes in biomarkers in individuals with these gene mutations and resulting disease variants will provide valuable insight into the specific changes that underlie the early events of onset of Alzheimer's disease. As an example, 15 years of study of a specific mutation in PSEN1 (where a single amino acid, number 280 in the protein sequence, is changed from glutamic acid to aspartic acid) revealed a consistent and predictable course of the disease that begins with mild cognitive impairment between 43–45 years of age and dementia by age 49–50. With such a specific timeline, dissecting out how the disease begins and defining the earliest biomarkers of the disease becomes more manageable.

The presenilins are actually a family of membrane proteins that serve as part of gamma-secretase. The presenilin component of gamma-secretase is the actual proteolytic entity; it is the enzymatic part that cleaves the remaining membrane-bound APP portion to release the amyloid beta peptide. Humans have two presenilin genes: PSEN1 and PSEN2 that code for presenilin-1 and presenilin-2, respectively. Either of these two closely related presenilins can contribute to gamma-secretase but presenilin-1 is the main cause of early-onset familial Alzheimer's disease. The mutations that occur in the genes lead to amino acid changes in the proteins, as summarized in Figure 12.3. Only 15 mutations in PSEN2 have been linked to familial Alzheimer's. In contrast, over 160 rare mutations in PSEN1 have been linked to this form of the disease. Each of these PSEN1 mutations results in a defined pattern of plaque formation and resultant effects. In total, the PSEN1 mutations are responsible for 70% of familial Alzheimer's disease and thus are the most common cause of it.

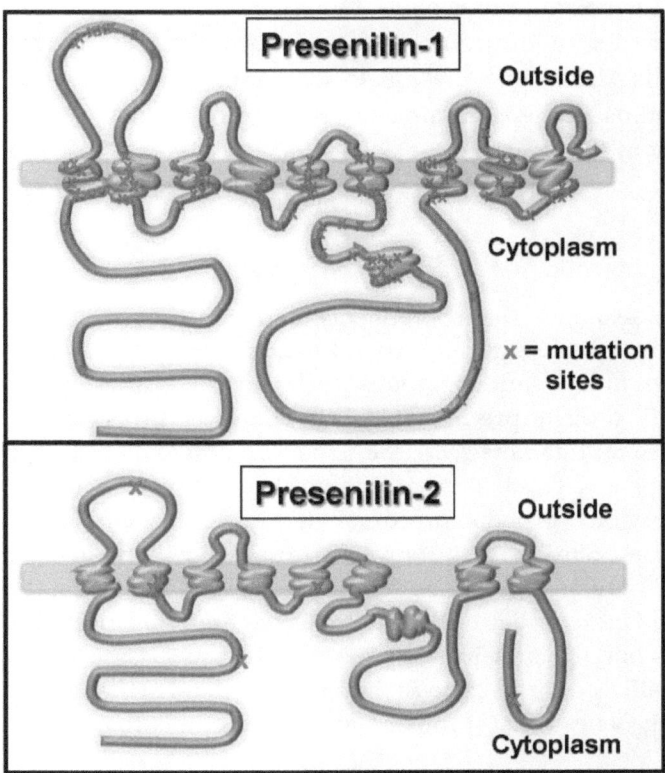

Figure 12.3. The mutation sites (red x's) of presenilin-1 and presenilin-2. Note how most of the presenilin-1 mutations are clustered primarily within amino acids inside the membrane (blue line).

Certain mutations in the gene alter the way gamma-secretase processes the remaining membrane-bound fragment of APP after beta-secretase action. Normal gamma-secretase produces more

Aβ40 than Aβ42. Certain APP mutations instead cause the release of larger amounts of the more amyloidogenic Aβ42 form of the peptide. Recent research has shown that presenilin also is involved in protein turnover which refers to the removal of unwanted, excess or no longer useful proteins and peptides. As such, presenilins also serve to specifically remove excess amyloid beta. When presenilins are mutated, they cannot break down amyloid thus allowing the peptide to build up to levels which promote plaque formation. Thus, individuals with PSEN1 or PSEN2 gene mutations show higher levels of Aβ42 versus Aβ40 and greater amounts of senile plaques than those who have sporadic Alzheimer's disease. Research into using drugs targeting presenilins, called gamma-secretase modulators, is currently underway.

* * *

FYI: Clarification of Terminology

As we examine the components and function of the gamma-secretase complex, it's important to again address the way they are referred to by various groups and journals. Earlier we covered amyloid protein precursor (APP), which is processed by beta-secretase and gamma-secretase to release amyloid beta peptides. If this were a scientific journal it might be more correct to write it as beta-amyloid protein precursor (βAPP) or β-amyloid protein precursor. Similarly, the proteins presenilin-1 (PSEN1) and -2 (PSEN2) are sometimes written as PS1 and PS2. It would also be appropriate to italicize these terms if we are referring to the genes that encode the proteins. That's how scientists clarify if the protein (non-italicized) or its gene (italicized) is under discussion (See, "FYI: Naming Genes versus Proteins" at the start of this chapter).

APOE is the short form for the protein apolipoprotein E but sometimes it is written apoE. Of course, there are usually many variants of genes that encode our proteins and APOE is no exception since it exists in three major forms. Without getting too bogged down in terminology, for Alzheimer's disease the E4 form of the apolipoprotein E gene is the one linked to the early onset of the disease. Thus its short form is APOE4 or ApoE4 although more formally the E is replaced by the Greek symbol for Epsilon.

* * *

The value of studying this specific mutation was evident in a study published at the end of 2012 in Lancet Neurology. As mentioned throughout this volume and detailed in Chapter 6, the accumulation of amyloid plaques is a cardinal neuropathological feature of Alzheimer's disease that is linked to both neuronal miscommunication and cell death. Using an amyloid-specific dye and PET imaging, it was found that amyloid beta accumulation in the cortex of the brain of individuals with a PSEN1 gene mutation was evident 16 years prior to the onset of mild cognitive impairment and 21 years prior to dementia. Thus, at least for this form of early-onset Alzheimer's disease, a more precise timeline was presented for the appearance of amyloid beta and its relationship to onset of the disease.

However, by the design of the experiments, which involved analyzing individuals at one point in their lives, it is possible that amyloid beta accumulation may actually occur even earlier. It's even possible it may begin to appear and increase in amount starting at birth. That remains to be studied. While some researchers suggest caution in interpreting the results, this information gives new insight into the earliest phases of the disease and may direct how future pharmaceutical trials linked to stopping the progression of the disease will be designed.

Some Good News: Gene Mutation Defends Against Alzheimer's

A 2012 study of 1,795 Icelanders led to an amazing discovery. A single point mutation in the amyloid precursor protein (APP) gene which resulted in a change in one amino acid in the amyloid precursor protein provided protection against developing Alzheimer's disease. This protein can consist of up to 770 amino acids, so the single mutation represents only 0.13% of the protein. However, this single amino acid change is sufficient to protect a person from getting the disease. How does it do this?

The single amino acid change resides in the region of amyloid precursor protein where beta-secretase cuts it. Because of this change, the enzyme cannot recognize this region and, thus, can't chop off the soluble amyloid precursor protein (sAPP). As a result, the amyloid beta-containing fragment is not available for release by the action of gamma-secretase.

Those results revealed that only 0.5% of Icelanders have this protective mutation. Those who do have the mutation are five times more likely to grow old without getting Alzheimer's. In addition, around 0.2–0.5% of Finns, Norwegians and Swedes also possess the mutated gene. While these low numbers might not seem that impressive, there is an additional silver lining to the APP mutant cloud. The first is that this work strongly supports other research linking amyloid beta with Alzheimer's disease. The second is it unequivocally strengthens the view that inhibiting beta-secretase function is a viable route to pursue. In fact several pharmaceutical companies have developed beta-secretase inhibitors that are now in clinical trials. While previous work with such inhibitors has not been successful, this new research suggests that continuing to look for agents that shut down beta-secretase and hence stop or slow amyloid beta formation is a worthy goal.

Late-Onset Susceptibility Genes

Most of the genetic basis associated with late-onset Alzheimer's is due to the action of multiple genes without a clearly defined pattern of inheritance. As a result they are considered to be susceptibility genes rather than genes that directly cause Alzheimer's. Because these genes are risk factors rather than causes it hasn't been easy to find them. After all, not all who suffer from Alzheimer's disease have the exact same disease or symptoms. There are also differences based on genetic backgrounds and nationality, among other factors. Thus finding late-onset susceptibility genes required complex statistical analyses, called meta-analysis, coupled with Genome-Wide Association Study (GWAS) carried out by researchers in the various international Alzheimer's disease consortia.

To date, only 14 genes have shown a strong relationship to Alzheimer's disease. Having specific mutations in these genes is a risk factor and not a more direct cause, as we saw with early-onset Alzheimer's disease. While the presence of mutations in these genes is linked to Alzheimer's disease, the relationship to the disease for many of them still is under analysis. We'll first look at the genes that have been identified that are intimately tied to the formation and turnover of amyloid beta. Then we will examine some of the newly identified genes that seem to cause Alzheimer's disease by less obvious routes.

The first genetic analyses identified an Alzheimer's disease triumvirate: three genes that were known to be linked as rare causes of early-onset Alzheimer's disease: APP, PSEN1 and PSEN2. Subsequent research identified a fourth gene that also could lead to late-onset Alzheimer's disease. Specifically, the epsilon4 form of the APOE gene, which encodes apolipoprotein E, is a strong risk factor for Alzheimer's disease. This form of the gene was also mentioned in the subsection, "FYI: Clarification of Terminology". Hereafter, we'll generally refer to it simply as APOE.

The discovery of APOE was followed by the identification of Alzheimer's disease risk factor gene number five, a gene called SORL1. Adding to what may appear to be an increasing and meaningless list of alphanumerics, nine more genes have been added to the susceptibility gene profile: ABCA7, BIN1, CD33, CD2AP, CLU, CR1, EPHA1, MS4A4E/MS4A6A and PICALM. That number will likely increase.

So what do we know about all of these genetic suspects as potential risk factors for developing Alzheimer's disease? Are their names just random jumbles of letters that sprung from scientific database analyses? Or do the names mean something that relates directly to how Alzheimer's disease occurs and progresses? Do these genes have any relationship to the hallmarks of the disease, amyloid plaques and tangles? Or do they open up new, previously unknown pathways to understanding the disease? Let's begin answering these questions by looking at those genes that are linked to amyloid plaque formation.

Good Genes Can Do Bad Things

It can be confusing to scientists when they find that a certain molecule with a defined cellular function actually does many other things. The common rule for cell proteins is that they have more than one job. Since there are only around 25,000 functional genes in cells, it is imperative that the encoded proteins serve many different roles. This is true for the protein encoded by the APOE gene. This gene codes for the protein apolipoprotein E

(APOE). APOE is involved in lipid metabolism, specifically cholesterol transport. In the brain this function is important in forming the connections between neurons (i.e., synaptogenesis — the formation of synapses) which is critical for brain cell communication and thus underlies all brain functions. There is also evidence APOE binds amyloid beta to prevent its incorporation into plaques and/or lead to its uptake into cells by endocytosis. While all of these functions are possible, the actual role of APOE in Alzheimer's disease is unknown.

APOE: A Cholesterol-Associated Protein Linked to Alzheimer's

Apolipoprotein E is a protein that can combine with lipids (fats) in the body to form lipoproteins. Normally fats are not soluble in aqueous environments like the blood. This biochemical packaging as lipoproteins allows the fats to be transported in the blood. Low-density lipoproteins (LDLs) are used to transport cholesterol. APOE is a predominant component of very low-density lipoproteins (vLDLs) which function in transporting cholesterol to the liver where it can be processed.

The APOE gene, as its name implies, encodes the APOE protein. There are more than three forms of the gene, or what geneticists call alleles. Of these, there are three major forms referred to as e2, e3 and e4. Many diseases and disorders are linked to these gene variants including atherosclerosis (APOE e4), hyperlipoproteinemia (APOE e2) and macular degeneration (APOE e2). APOE e4 is of interest here because it has been linked to an increased risk of forming amyloid plaques and of developing late-onset Alzheimer's disease. Individuals who inherit a single copy of the APOE e4 form of the gene have an increased chance of being affected by the disease. Two copies of the gene further increase the risk of Alzheimer's disease. That said, it is important to note that a person having the APOE e4 form of the gene does not mean they will suffer from the disease. Also, not everyone who has Alzheimer's has the APOE e4 gene.

* * *

Interesting Factoids: APOE e4

The APOE e4 form of the apolipoprotein E gene also increases the risk for dementia in people who have Parkinson's disease.

When does APOE e4 have its effect? Recent research indicates that mutations in this gene affect the brain at birth, which suggests that this form of the gene may begin having its negative effects during fetal development.

* * *

APOE is known to act as a dose-dependent factor in developing Alzheimer's disease. Individuals from different ethnic populations possess different levels of the e4 allele of the gene. The e4 allele specifically decreases the age at which Alzheimer's onset occurs from 84 to 68 years of age. It also increases the risk of developing Alzheimer's from 20% to 90%. As we have seen, APOE is also linked to the onset and progression of Alzheimer's disease in Down syndrome individuals but not in people who develop the early-onset form of the disease. In late-onset Alzheimer's disease, APOE is found in senile plaques and is linked to amyloid beta deposition and clearance in the brain. In spite of all this, APOE apparently does not work alone. APOE is not required for the development of Alzheimer's disease nor is it sufficient to cause the disease. As a result, it was hoped that Genome-Wide Association Studies would add insight into the situation. This information is discussed in the next chapter.

Chapter 13

More Susceptibility Genes

Alzheimer's disease may best be described as a syndrome. This is because there are at least three distinct types: Down syndrome, early-onset and late-onset Alzheimer's disease. Each of these has a distinct genetic profile as detailed previously. As a result the signs and symptoms of the disease are also variable, even within each of these three general types. Given that Alzheimer's may in fact represent a syndrome with multiple variable causes, it's not unexpected then that multiple genes are linked to the disease both as risk and susceptibility genes, if not direct causes. Here we will look at some of the newer genetic players associated with late-onset Alzheimer's disease. We will also introduce the area of Genome-Wide Association Studies (GWAS) that is revealing the precise mutations linked to Alzheimer's and may in the future forge the way for precise genetic testing as the search for the causes and a cure continues.

Putting Amyloid Beta in the Garbage Instead of in Plaques

While humans have only recently caught on to the value of recycling, this process has been essential for the growth and survival of cells. No molecule lasts forever in normal cells. New molecules are made and old ones turned over so their components can be recycled for other uses. The same goes for amyloid beta. The peptide is produced and it is recycled. The amount of peptide that is present in any one place at any time is due to the amount of its synthesis versus the amount of its recycling. One of the genes involved in the recycling of amyloid beta is the gene called SORL1.

SORL1 encodes a receptor that is involved in the movement of vesicles from the cell membrane to the inside of the cell where any contained molecules can be modified or broken down. When the vesicles contain amyloid precursor protein (APP), this affects the processing of the protein and as a result the production of amyloid beta. Thus SORL1 is a risk gene because mutations that inhibit its ability to assist in recycling amyloid beta mean more of the peptide remains outside of the cell for plaque formation. That said, this working hypothesis is just that: an idea yet to be proven.

Nine Offenders with Unfriendly Names

Genome-Wide Association Studies have identified numerous risk genes, of which nine stand out. Our goal here is to summarize them because the identified genes and potential therapies linked to them are less on the forefront than those involving other genes and specific target proteins. It would have been helpful if only a couple of genes were linked to the development of late-onset Alzheimer's disease but that's not the case. After all, some diseases have been linked to mutations in a single protein. For example, Tay-Sachs disease is caused by the loss or malfunction of a single enzyme, hexosaminidase A. With such diseases cures can be found, such as enzyme or gene replacement among other therapies. But when many genes are involved, as typifies cancer and Alzheimer's disease, then the search for causes and a cure becomes much more complex.

As mentioned above, the genes are an alphanumeric conglomerate that few will remember: ABCA7, BIN1, CD33, CD2AP, CLU, CR1, EPHA1, MS4A4E/MS4A6A and PICALM. While they are not names to remember, their link to Alzheimer's disease makes them worthy of some attention. Each of the letters in the genes, as we will see, refers to the known protein encoded by the gene. Here we will simply outline what proteins each of these genes encodes and then we'll try to tie all this apparent genetic mess into a coherent picture—it won't be an easy task.

ABCA7 stands for the mouth-filling term "ATP-binding cassette transporter member 7" which is not as easy to learn as your real ABC's. The ABC transporters have a long evolutionary history, being present from early bacteria to humans. Usually such evolutionary conservation suggests fundamentally important proteins in cell function. ATP-binding cassette transporters, as their name suggests, use the energy stored in ATP to transport or move various molecules, including drugs, across membranes at the surface and inside of cells. They are linked to cystic fibrosis and cancer among a host of other human diseases. They are also involved in the development of resistance to drugs. While a large amount is known about ABC transporters, their role in Alzheimer's disease remains enigmatic.

BIN1 is the short form for bridging integrator protein 1. While there is strong evidence that this protein is a risk factor for Alzheimer's, how it is implicated remains to be determined. In fact, comparatively little is really known about BIN1. It may be involved in transporting materials across membranes and it may act as a tumor suppressor. There is evidence it functions in muscle contraction and mutations in the protein can cause certain muscle diseases. Without more pure research on the protein, it is difficult to know how it is involved in Alzheimer's disease or how it can be used as a pharmaceutical target.

CD33 doesn't have another name and isn't an acronym for anything. It is a gene linked to the immune system where it codes for a membrane immune receptor protein. It affects cell proliferation of myeloid cells but its role in the brain is unknown.

CD2AP refers to CD2-associated protein, a protein that acts as scaffolding for the cell's cytoskeleton. Specifically associating with filamentous actin, it can affect how the membrane works during cell division, endocytosis and organizing a cell's shape. Mutations in the gene have been liked to kidney disease. The protein has been studied for over a decade but its role in Alzheimer's disease remains to be revealed.

CLU is the gene encoding the protein clusterin which is also known as apolipoprotein J (APOJ). It is involved in membrane recycling, cell adhesion and controlling cell death. While a diversity of studies have linked clusterin/APOJ to Alzheimer's, its mode of action is unclear.

CR1, or complement receptor type 1, encodes a membrane protein involved in the immune response. It mediates the binding between particles and activated immune cells. Reduced levels of the protein are linked to lupus erythematosus, HIV infection and certain anemias. Ongoing research suggests that CR1's involvement in Alzheimer's disease is linked to its role in the immune response.

EPHA1, or ephrin receptor A1, is a protein that regulates the pattern of growth of neurons, guiding them in the right direction to form appropriate contacts with other nerve cells or specific tissues. These receptors are kinases that are also involved in limb development, the formation of the blood system and cancer.

MS4A4E and **MS4A6A** are acronyms for two variants of membrane-spanning 4-domains subfamily A, member 4E and member 6A, respectively. These variants were only recently linked to late-onset Alzheimer's by three independent research groups. While the encoded proteins have not been well characterized, there is evidence they function in the immune response and possibly form ion channels in the membranes of non-immune cell types.

PICALM is the short form for the mouthful "phosphatidylinositol-binding clathrin assembly protein". This protein binds to certain lipids, called phosphatidylinositols, in the cell membrane where they recruit a specific protein (i.e., clathrin) that is involved in endocytosis. The role of this protein in Alzheimer's disease has not yet been revealed.

PICALM Stands Out in One Study

A paper detailing the statistical analysis of 701 Alzheimer's patients with specific gene mutations linked to the disease via Genome-Wide Association Studies was reported at the start of 2013. Of the genes studied—APOE and six others (five mentioned above: CLU, PICALM, CR1, BIN1, MS4A; and EXOC3L2)—only PICALM showed any statistically significant relationship to the onset and progression of the disease. Clearly genetics, lifestyle and environment work in complex ways to define Alzheimer's. These and other kinds of comparative genetic studies should ultimately shed detailed light on the genes and how lifestyle and the environment work with them to induce the disease.

GWAS: Genome-Wide Association Studies

Although the majority of those with Alzheimer's disease exhibit the late-onset form of the disease, finding the genes responsible has been extremely challenging. However, a multitude of Genome-Wide Association Studies have begun to provide some insight, if not the answer we need. Over a dozen different groups worldwide are involved in GWAS. They have studied millions of potential gene mutations in thousands of Alzheimer's sufferers as well as in non-Alzheimer's individuals (which serve as controls). They primarily use markers called single-nucleotide polymorphisms (SNPs, pronounced "snips"). SNPs are single-nucleotide (base) changes in the DNA which differ in different individuals and even in the paired chromosomes of a single person.

* * *

FYI: SNPing Alzheimer's Disease

If you've had some high school or college/university science or watched science shows on TV, you'll probably remember DNA is made up of nucleotides (or, DNA bases). There are only four bases in DNA: G = Guanine, C = Cytosine, A = Adenine, T = Thymine. Each three bases can code for a specific amino acid in a protein. So if you change the bases in the DNA, you can change the amino acids they code for. Since proteins are made up of amino acids, when you change one amino acid it can seriously affect how that protein folds and how it functions. An example of an SNP (pronounced "snip") could be a change from CGAGATTCG to CGAGATTTG. If the amino acid specified by this region was critical to the function of the protein in question and if this protein was linked to a disease, then this SNP could be important for detecting that disease.

* * *

Less often, researchers have used Copy Number Variations (CNVs) to see if there are genes linked to late-onset Alzheimer's disease. In this instance, there has been an increase or decrease in the number of copies for a specific gene. We mentioned previously that trisomy 21 or Down syndrome individuals have an extra chromosome 21. While this is a whole chromosome it can be used to understand the effect of additional copies of a gene. In this case, there are extra copies of all of the genes on chromosome 21. So having extra genes, such as the amyloid protein precursor gene, which are correlated with a risk of Alzheimer's disease will increase the chance that person will develop the disease.

Finding the gene alterations that are linked to Alzheimer's disease is made possible by comparing gene sequences of non-Alzheimer's individuals with those who have the disease. Selection of Alzheimer's disease and control (normal) individuals for such studies is based on cognitive testing or magnetic resonance imaging, to name two major testing schemes. Groups can also be selected or sub-grouped based on other factors including family history, country, ethnicity and ancestry. For example, there are more cases of Alzheimer's disease worldwide among Europeans and Asians than other groups. Studying individuals from diverse backgrounds thus can provide useful insight into other contributing factors (e.g., diet, environment, etc.), not only the genes responsible for late-onset Alzheimer's disease.

To date, using GWAS studies has revealed more than twenty genes that are linked to late-onset Alzheimer's disease. Of these, one gene shows what some consider an unequivocal relationship with late-onset Alzheimer's disease: APOE. But as discussed below, APOE cannot alone be the cause of the disease and it is not essential for the development of the late-onset form of the disease. Of the other dozens of proteins linked to Alzheimer's, many appear consistently in all of the different studies. For example, acetylcholinesterase (AChE), discussed in Chapter 9, has been of interest and is a target for various Alzheimer's therapies.

In spite of having identified various risk genes, their potential to be the cause of Alzheimer's disease, either alone or in concert with other suspect proteins, is minimal. That said, it is possible that the link between these suspect proteins is not a simple paired or group interaction but a complex higher level of multiple interactions. The issue of epigenetic gene modifications is also a possibility, as discussed below. In short, attempts to find a hereditary link between genes and the development of late-onset Alzheimer's disease have not identified the culprit involved.

While the results from such research are frustrating, they are still fruitful because they provide insight and guidance to carry research forward in other potentially productive areas. For example, many of the implicated genes have been shown to possess specific mutations which were linked to Alzheimer's disease. However, the gene mutations that were found in different groups and individuals were unique. There was no single mutation that could be linked to the disease. Further GWAS studies on larger groups of individuals with specific focus on ethnicity and ancestry may yield additional insight. The key with such studies is that even results that appear negative are in many ways useful and essential because they guide the next phases of research.

If you are interested, you can keep up on the progress of the GWAS studies at the Alzgene website (www.alzgene.org). A multitude of other resources are there as well. But the site is mainly designed to assist workers in the field, as opposed to the layperson with no scientific background.

* * *

FYI: Alzheimer's Beyond the Gene

One of the hottest areas of research in the life and biomedical sciences these days is epigenetics. This literally means above ("epi") the gene ("genetics"). In layperson's terms, these are chemical changes made to the DNA of our genome that are in addition to the actual gene sequences. These chemical changes define how the genetic information is read in different cells at different times. All genes are encoded in four bases: adenine (A), cytosine (C), guanine (G) and thymine (T). (One of my friends uses the acronym GCAT for "George CAT" to help students remember.) Extended sequences of these four bases spell out our genes and these are passed on from generation to generation. Mutations can be caused by many events and these can be passed on. The way genes are read (transcribed) and/or silenced (not transcribed) is regulated by other genes and regulatory sequences in our genome. But there is more.

Our genes can also be modified by some of the processes that also affect how our proteins function. We've already seen how phosphorylation and dephosphorylation regulate normal protein function in the case of tau—protein hyperphosphorylation turns this good protein bad. There are other protein-modifying events as well including methylation, acetylation and ubiquination, to mention the most widely studied. Interestingly, these same modifications can be done to our DNA—and then they can be passed on to our children. So what does this have to do with Alzheimer's disease?

The study of epigenetic modifications has only recently become a focus in Alzheimer's disease. Epigenetics provide a mechanism whereby environmental factors can influence how genes are expressed and silenced. A diversity of factors including diet, smoking, UV exposure and other hazardous life events can lead to alterations in our genes, some of which are also linked to the onset and progression of Alzheimer's disease.

The area of focus so far has been on DNA methylation but so far it is only in its infancy. One study has shown that DNA methylation was decreased in seven specific genes in cortical neurons and glia but not in other brain regions in individuals with the disease. Studies using APP mouse models have also shown similar results. The potential importance of epigenetic regulation of Alzheimer's disease is also suggested by the fact APP, BACE, and PSEN1, which were discussed in Chapter 12, all possess methylated gene sites.

To take this one step further, experiments have shown that treatments with amyloid beta induced decreased global methylation of genes in the brains of mice and human cells in culture. Interestingly, while the majority of genes had low levels of methylation (i.e., were hypomethylated), the gene for neprilysin, an amyloid beta-degrading enzyme, had high levels of methylation (i.e., was hypermethylated). This and other work strongly suggests that epigenetic mechanisms involving gene methylation are linked to Alzheimer's disease.

Future studies similar to GWAS are required to assess the relationship of specific gene methylation with the onset and progression of Alzheimer's disease. This might be the key that opens the box of understanding of the results from genome-wide studies. Maybe it's not the specific gene mutations in APOE or in the other suspect Alzheimer's susceptibility proteins but in their epigenetic modifications. Once that is understood, the next step would be to determine what causes these epigenetic modifications. The search for the cause of Alzheimer's disease will be long a one. As new areas of research like this open up they offer concrete hope for the future.

* * *

Chapter 14

Developing a Drug Takes Time

Current medical interventions for Alzheimer's disease are designed to provide symptomatic relief, not cure the disease. In Chapters 9 and 10, we discussed some of the other pharmaceutical approaches that are used with a focus on the two most significant: cholinesterase inhibitors and NMDA antagonists. To date, however, the vast majority of research has focused on the "amyloid cascade hypothesis". As mentioned in Chapter 8, this dominant hypothesis is based on data indicating that the enzymatic processing of amyloid protein precursor into neurotoxic amyloid beta peptides is central to the etiopathology of the disease. Since this approach dominates the pharmacological approaches aimed at the management of Alzheimer's disease, we will begin with this topic. When that's done, we'll take a quick look at some of the new therapies that are being explored. In each case, we'll set the stage with background about the drug targets and how they function in normal cells.

It's important to note that scientists studying Alzheimer's are faced with a significant problem. Whenever a biological system is compromised, in addition to the primary and secondary effects, there are also lots of changes that are not specifically related to the issue at hand. In other words, when any disease strikes it throws off the basic balance (homeostasis) of other systems in the body. This usually has serious effects on these other non-target systems. In simple terms, scientists, like detectives, must find the actual cause while trying to avoid these "red herrings" that distract and confuse the search.

Dealing with Symptoms versus Causes

Historically, treatments for Alzheimer's disease have been designed to slow the progression of the disease so that life gets better for the person coping with the disease and his or her caregivers. In short, a great deal of Alzheimer's drug development has been designed to deal with the symptoms, not the causes of the disease.

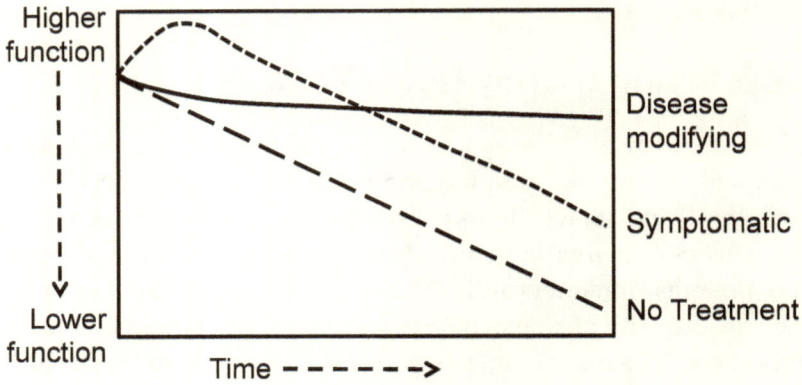

Figure 14.1. The time course of loss of higher brain function with disease-modifying treatment, treatment for symptomatic conditions and in the absence of treatment. (After Figure 1 in Vellas et al., 2011. Alzheimer's & Dementia 7: e109–e117)

As shown in Figure 14.1, with time the individual suffering from Alzheimer's will experience a steady decline in cognitive and social function when no treatment is used or available. As its name implies, the symptomatic approach deals with therapies that are aimed at alleviating the symptoms of the disease. The symptomatic approach can lead to significant short-term improvement which is then usually followed by a steady but continual loss of function. Thus, while there is clear initial improvement in symptoms, there is no real rescue from the ultimate fate facing the Alzheimer's sufferer. The third approach is to deal with the development and progress of the disease itself. With the disease-modifying approach, the progress of the disease may be stopped in its tracks. This is the primary goal of research today since by slowing or stopping the progression of the disease there will be coincident alleviation of the symptoms associated with it.

Why is it Taking So Long?

In spite of the significance of Alzheimer's disease to society, families and the individual, one might think there has been little progress made in finding ways to slow or stop the disease, let alone prevent it. There are many reasons that a viable drug has not been forthcoming and why an effective one may not be developed for many years to come. First, the actual "cause" of Alzheimer's disease is still unknown. The search for this cause is being done by a multitude of dedicated scientists worldwide but this is not an easy task. Based on the variability of the disease characteristics from person to person, there likely isn't a single cause. In addition, neurons in the brain, like all human cells, are very complex biological systems that still aren't understood completely. After all, if we don't understand all of the normal workings of a cell, how can we hope to truly understand what goes wrong in a diseased cell? That said, appropriate scientific tinkering can still lead to important insights and pharmaceutical development in the absence of a full understanding of how and why those drugs are effective. The aforementioned issues can also be applied to the development of drugs that can slow or stop the progression of Alzheimer's disease from mild cognitive impairment to dementia. While some major players, including amyloid plaque and neurofibrillary tangle formation, have been identified the exact steps in the process still remain a mystery. More to the point, it is only recently that societies whose goal is to find cures for Alzheimer's disease have begun to clarify exactly how each stage in the development of the disease should be defined and characterized.

How can you prescribe the appropriate drug if you haven't got a handle on exactly what you are attempting to prevent, stop or cure? A great stride has been made in the cure for breast cancer as well as other cancers. By genetic screening and tumor profiling, scientists can now apply drug regimens that are individual and cancer specific. While in the past drugs like tamoxifen were used as a general therapeutic approach, it is now clear that this drug only works in specific cases. Now with cancer profiling, an appropriate drug regimen can be developed that targets the specific tumor and is, thus, more effective. Already combinatorial drug regimens are being tested for slowing the progression of Alzheimer's but as yet profiling is an unfulfilled dream because we don't understand it as well as we will in the future.

To summarize, we need to understand the actual initial cellular changes that transform normal brain cells into future Alzheimer's brain cells. As we have seen, there are a multitude of approaches that are being taken. For example, they focus on oxidative stress, calcium levels, and inflammatory responses which in turn can lead to amyloid plaque formation and neurofibrillary tangle production. Other psychological and biomedical biomarkers are also being developed so that the earliest stages of the disease can be estimated, allowing early intervention. Adding to this is another delaying factor: the time it takes to develop the drug for actual human use.

Stages of Drug Development

Once the cause or causes of Alzheimer's are identified, then it will be possible to develop pharmaceuticals to prevent the onset of the disease. Before this, it is more likely that drugs that slow or stop the disease will be developed. Even then, it is a long road from finding a pharmaceutical target to the actual appearance of such drugs in the marketplace. On average it takes from 10 to 15 years to develop a pharmaceutical. Thus, if a cause of Alzheimer's was discovered in 2015, we would not expect to see a cause-specific drug on the market until sometime between 2025 and 2030.

A similar scenario applies to understanding how Alzheimer's disease progresses since, again, a decade or more would be required to get a drug based on this to market. Of course, finding a way to slow the disease or prevent it will be a major boon to society and to younger individuals who haven't yet developed the disease, but it is of little solace to those currently fighting Alzheimer's. So why does it take so long? This is because there are specific stages in drug development that must be followed before human use is permitted. These are summarized in the following chart (Figure 14.2) and discussed below.

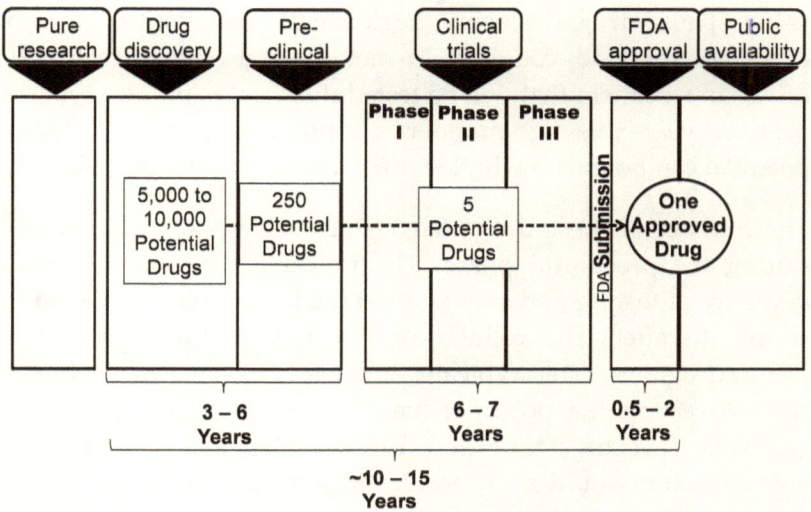

Figure 14.2. The stages in developing an Alzheimer's drug, from pure research to public availability.
(Modified from the article "Drug discovery and development" by the Pharmaceutical Research and Manufacturers of America, 2007)

The initial phase in the development of any drug typically results from pure research. It may be hard to believe but without basic scientific research aimed a simply understanding how things work, then the vast majority of drugs on the market would not exist. For example, penicillin was discovered through pure research by the Scottish biologist Sir Alexander Fleming when he noticed that bacteria couldn't grow around the mold *Penicillium notatum*. There are multitudes of examples of such discoveries that have changed the course of human history and medicine that were not discovered by doctors or pharmaceutical companies but by basic scientists trying to understand how things work. Sadly, this aspect of scientific research is quickly being phased out.

But let's assume some potential useful compounds have been discovered through years or decades of pure research and focus on the timeline for development of an effective Alzheimer's drug. Today new approaches have been developed that allow researchers to design variants of potentially effective compounds, enhancing the chances of finding at least one with downstream therapeutic value. Thus, drug discovery begins with the identification of effective compounds coupled with methods that generate thousands of variants of them that will be tested during this phase. Over the next few years this high number of approximately 5,000 to 10,000 potential compounds is whittled down to a couple of hundred or so.

The number of these drugs (e.g., ~250) will get further reduced during the preclinical phase. The preclinical phase involves a diversity of testing and evaluation. First the compound has to be shown to affect the cellular or biochemical target that it is directed against. This typically involves biochemical testing as well as testing the potential harmful effects of the drugs. For example if cells are killed by the drug, the compound automatically would be rejected. After testing in tissue culture, animal testing is done. Various Alzheimer's disease animal models exist but most commonly this involves different types of mouse strains, including some with Alzheimer's-related attributes. If the drug is effective in animal models and has few if any side effects of concern, then the drug is ready for human testing. Thus after over three to six years of testing in the drug discovery and preclinical stages, only a handful of potentially effective drugs will make it to the clinical trials stage.

The clinical trials stage involves human testing, first with small groups of volunteers and finally with large numbers that permit detailed statistical evaluation of the drug's efficacy. During Phase I of the clinical trials, the remaining five or so potential drugs that survived the preclinical evaluation in our example are tested on a small group (e.g., 20–100) of volunteer individuals. Since this small test group requires that in addition to individuals with Alzheimer's an appropriate number of control subjects (people without the disease). As a result, due to small numbers these preliminary results often give tentative but not reliable results due to statistical error. Thus any drug that might appear successful still remains in question because of the small number of test subjects in the trial. However, any compounds that do generate interesting results are subsequently tested on a larger (e.g., 100–500) volunteer group during Phase II trials where appropriate statistical analysis of the data is possible.

Finally, compounds that make the cut are tested on a significantly greater population of volunteers (e.g., 1000–5000). If all goes well, and that's no guarantee because of all of the other issues that arise (e.g., toxicity, deleterious side effects, ineffectiveness, etc.), at best one drug might survive the clinical stages. After documenting the results and submission to the FDA in the US, or the appropriate drug administration body in other countries, the drug may or may not get approval after up to two years of review. With approval, the pharmaceutical companies kick their drug production into high gear, putting the drug on the market and promoting it with the knowledge that time is a factor in getting the drug to market and keeping it there as long as possible.

Thus we can see that getting from drug discovery to market is a complex and involved process. While families, individuals and society might be frustrated by the lack of appropriate Alzheimer's drug development, it is an arduous process that still suffers from our not having full understanding of the causes of the disease and the actual sequence of events that leads from mild cognitive impairment to full-blown dementia.

Scientist versus Clinician versus Patient: Different Points of View

The doctor or scientist who is studying Alzheimer's disease and/or trying to find a drug to combat the disease often has to view his or her data in a different light than those coping with the disease and their caregivers. Those searching for effective drugs have to assess their success based upon statistical analysis of the data that is generated in clinical trials. So the goal of these trials boils down to getting a statistically significant positive outcome. Results that are statistically significant mean that the drug's effect is mathematically different from that to which the drug (e.g., placebo, drug variant) is compared. So the criteria can be different than the Alzheimer's individual or their caregivers want or need. Also, a small statistical effect may not be of real significance in treating the symptoms or progression of the disease. This may be due to an unacceptable cost of using the drug in any therapy or the existence of serious side effects.

This brings us into the realm of clinical significance. Here large differences need to be validated. Any drug that meets the definition of clinical significance must lead to major improvements that the doctor, patient and caregiver can see or feel. This analysis involves a risk versus cost versus benefit evaluation. These improvements must be enough to overcome any concerns about cost or side effects. Of course, while statistical significance is solid and based on real numbers, clinical significance involves the analysis of opinion, feelings and perceptions which then have to be interpreted into numbers that can be statistically analyzed. This is done through various assessment questions and psychological tests, among other things. Since success is in the eye of the beholder, it means different things to different people. In terms of Alzheimer's disease, improvement in social interactivity might hold more weight to one person or their caregiver while increased independence might suit others. We are all different and have different views on life—this doesn't change just because we have an affliction such as Alzheimer's disease.

But remember, opinions are just that. They are subjective and personal. This is why most meaningful clinical trials are double-blind experiments. Neither the patient nor the clinician knows who is getting what drug or placebo. When the data are analyzed, the statistician doesn't know what is being compared. It is only once the results of the study are complete and data are fully analyzed that drug and placebo groups are unmasked and significance or non-significance is realized. This procedure should be, and usually is, followed in each phase of clinical testing of a potential drug.

The Problems Facing Alzheimer's Drug Research

It's been pretty clear that Alzheimer's likely is not a simple disease with a single cause. This is only one problem facing Alzheimer's disease researchers. Many other issues come into play when doing pharmaceutical research. As discussed above, to obtain statistically significant results, studies need to involve a large number of individuals. You not only need those with the disease for testing both the drug and a placebo but you require healthy individuals as well. Selecting and classifying Alzheimer's individuals is not an easy task because of the variability in the disease. Also, the way the disease is categorized can vary depending on who is doing the categorization. Then the issue of education raises its head. Patients and their caregivers need to fully understand what they are getting into. The explanation of expectations and the patients' responsibilities must be made as clear as possible to those involved in the study. There must be no ambiguity or confusion. Of course, when people are involved on both sides of the issue, patients and their caregivers versus researchers and their assistants, there is always room for errors and confusion. Simply put, anything that involves a variety of people and complex information can quickly lead to confusion!

Once the study starts, there is attrition. As time passes, more and more individuals tend to drop out of Alzheimer's studies. Attrition is the bane of pharmaceutical research because it can really mess up the results. Participants leave for a number of reasons. For example, a person on a placebo who has Alzheimer's and who gets progressively and significantly worse is often at great risk of dropping out. With no progress, they feel it's a waste of time. Participants may also drop out because of lack of caregiver support. Without help, they may forget to take their medication regularly thus undermining analysis of the drug's effectiveness and making it invalid for them to continue in the study.

Attrition also results through death and as a result of individuals moving away so it is no longer convenient for them to continue in the study. At least one comprehensive analysis, reviewing approximately 60 other studies, revealed that the drug that was being investigated also affected patient dropout. Dropouts from the experimental groups (i.e., patients treated with the drug itself) were very much greater for acetylcholinesterase drug studies than for other drug studies such as those involving NMDA inhibitors. This has been suggested as being due to the fact that acetylcholinesterase inhibitors are more toxic, leading to greater side effects than occur with other Alzheimer's drugs. Often the types of individuals that drop out can skew the results by removing randomness. However, this problem can partly be overcome by proper experimental design and through the use of appropriate statistical analyses. For all of these and other reasons, attrition remains a continuing problem with such studies.

As a study progresses, some indication of the drug's effectiveness in individual patients will become evident as summarized in Figure 14.3. Often by six months, or some other predetermined time, an assessment will be made as to whether the subject involved shows a positive response to the drug, an indeterminate response or no response. At this point the patient will consult with his or her doctor or some other authorized individual to make a decision whether to continue with the same drug and treatment regimen, stop treatment or switch to another drug or treatment regimen. The arrows in the diagram below suggest the common routes that are followed.

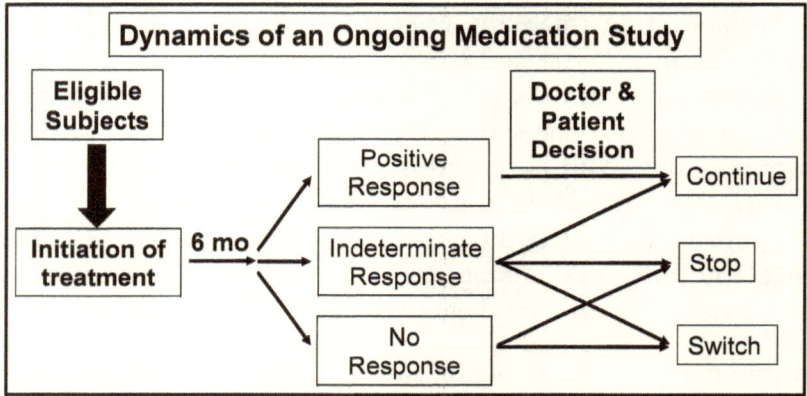

Figure 14.3. The dynamics of an ongoing medication study.

There are other aspects to Alzheimer's research that affect its progress. It costs a lot of money to carry out large clinical trials. This stems from the need for office space, computers and other things to facilitate the work of the large number of staff who collect, collate and analyze the data. True success also requires international collaboration which has its own issues in addition to needing sufficient funding. For example, cultural variations and differences can lead to variations in methodologies and approaches, which affect how the data can be analyzed and interpreted. This is just a sampling of the impediments such research faces.

So while the progress of research may seem slow at times, even negative results can be helpful. With the search for biomarkers in full stride, the future should provide more insight that will assist pharmaceutical companies in their quest for better drugs. Future progress will also lead to the development of patient-specific combinational therapies that will greatly increase chances to significantly slow the progression of the disease—if not stop it in its tracks.

Analyzing Drug Success Is an Issue

Once the study is done, the full data analysis begins. Many consider analysis to be the weak link in Alzheimer's disease drug studies for a number of reasons. Since people are a heterogeneous lot physically, physiologically and genetically, it is difficult at best to get any uniform and significant positive results. While all this might seem like much time has been wasted, there is a bright side. With Alzheimer's drugs, there have always been a few standout successes. Such results suggest that certain individuals respond favorably to drug treatments based on the status of their disease at the start, and/or genetics plus other reasons.

Thus, while statistically a drug might fail to help everyone, it may still help with a small cohort of people. This might be analogized to the situation with breast cancer. While certain breast cancer drugs help some women, they are no help to others and, in fact, may worsen the situation in some cases. As just one example, some breast cancer cells are very responsive to estrogen and will grow more actively in the presence of the hormone. Others are not responsive. So drugs that inhibit estrogen function will work in the former group but not the latter. Today, very complex genetic analyses are leading to treatments that are extremely patient specific. The goal of research is to do the same for Alzheimer's. So the search is on to understand this variability as it relates to Alzheimer's disease. Already, rather than simply providing a single pharmaceutical at a recommended dosage, drugs and drug regimens are being designed to meet specific aspects related to the individual.

A New Drug for Detecting Plaques

Typically, amyloid plaques are not revealed in the brain until autopsy. However, new imaging techniques have been developed to verify if amyloid deposits are present in the brain of living individuals. Let's look at a recent way that this is being done and the implications of this work. As a primary biomarker for Alzheimer's disease, the early detection of amyloid plaques in the brain is of central interest and of great focus in biomedical research. That interest was stimulated recently with the US Federal Drug Administration's approval of Amyvid™—the first and only radioactive diagnostic tool for the estimation of amyloid plaque density in people with cognitive impairment which could be a symptom of Alzheimer's disease. Amyvid™ is a product of Eli Lilly and Company and Avid Radiopharmaceuticals, a subsidiary of Eli Lilly. It is administered to patients by injection into a vein, and the localization of the radioactively labeled compound in the brain then is assessed by a PET (Positron Emission Tomography) scan.

Since Amyvid™ binds specifically to amyloid plaques, a negative result (little or no radioactive localization) indicates that the person does not have a significant level of plaque present in their brains. A positive result (lots of localized radioactivity), on the other hand indicates the presence of significant plaque buildup in the patient's brain. However, this alone is not proof of Alzheimer's disease because elderly individuals can have amyloid plaques in their brains but have normal cognitive function. That said, the presence of a positive Amyvid™ result coupled with other biomarkers such as impaired cognitive testing would strongly indicate the individual does have Alzheimer's. In short, on its own Amyvid™ is only one part of evaluating the presence of Alzheimer's disease.

At the moment, this is an expensive procedure for several reasons. First, the detector molecule Amyvid™ must be tagged with radioisotope fluorine-18 so it can be detected via PET scan. After Amyvid™ is produced it has to be radiolabeled locally because the fluorine label has a short half-life—its radioactivity is quickly lost. It only lasts a short period of time because half of its radioactivity is lost every two hours. So Amyvid™ must be bound to the isotope and then used in close proximity to where it was made so that it remains sensitive enough to be detected. The second expense-causing issue is that the results can only be interpreted properly by experts, usually radiologists who have been trained specifically to assess the results of the Amyvid™ PET scan. This leads into the third reason for the high cost: new readers have to be trained and approved. While these issues are being resolved quickly, it still means the assessment method will not be available in many areas for some time in the future.

It is also important to note that even though experts are trained in the diagnostic interpretation of the PET scan results with Amyvid™, errors can still result just as they can with any diagnostic procedure. So the level of error and success will only be revealed after extensive testing. Despite FDA approval, the long-term effects of administering Amyvid™ remain to be determined. At present however, it represents a significant step forward in evaluating the existence of amyloid buildup in the brain and, as such, may provide a valuable tool for Alzheimer's diagnosis in the long term.

While Amyvid™ is a way of assessing the presence of amyloid plaques that signal the existence of Alzheimer's disease, it is not a drug that offers any cure; only guidance and information. Pharmaceuticals that are currently being used to fight the symptoms of the disease, as well as routes to developing new drugs, are mentioned in various places and discussed in detail in Chapters 9 and 10. Since this is an ongoing, dynamic area, those who have specific interests should check out the various Alzheimer's organizations listed at the end of this book.

Chapter 15

The Pharmaceutical Landscape

A Timeline of Major Clinical Therapies

Figure 15.1 presents a timeline of the major avenues of Alzheimer's drug development. In Chapter 8, drugs that are linked to the amyloid hypothesis ("Amyloid drugs" in figure) were discussed. As indicated in the figure, this approach wasn't taken until around the turn of the century. The specific focus on secretases didn't begin until many years later. On the other hand, many other clinical therapies (e.g., acetylcholinesterase inhibitors, chelators, NMDA antagonists, etc.) had already been under investigation 10–20+ years prior to this.

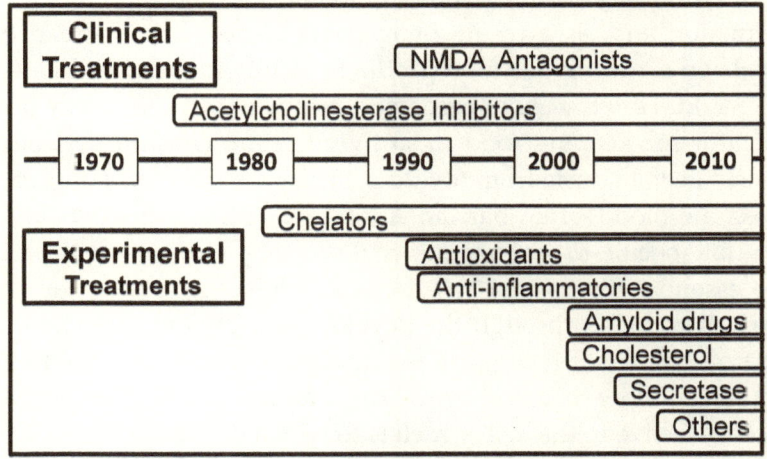

Figure 15.1. The timeline summarizing the major clinical therapies that have and are being used in the treatment of Alzheimer's disease. (Modified from Figure 1 in Stone et al., 2011)

Two of the most intensely studied areas are acetylcholinesterase inhibitors and NMDA antagonists. These were covered in Chapters 9 and 10, respectively. Historically the earliest research was aimed at acetylcholinesterase inhibitors starting in the 1970s while NMDA antagonists became a target beginning around the 1990s.

Of these two clinical treatments, the development and use of acetylcholinesterase inhibitors has a comparatively long history because acetylcholine is well known as a critical brain molecule involved in nerve cell communication. Thus even today and into the future, acetylcholinesterase inhibitors will be used and new pharmaceuticals based on this approach will be developed. This chapter will delve into some detail on the work done on several other treatments (e.g., antioxidants, anti-inflammatories, cholesterol drugs).

Chelation Therapy

On the experimental side, studies with chelators have been on the books since the early 1980s but for the most part these haven't led to effective therapies. Copper and iron levels are elevated in Alzheimer's brains where they play a part in the assembly of amyloid beta to form amyloid plaques. Chelating agents can bind to these heavy metals, making them unavailable for plaque formation and, as a result, neurodegeneration. (If you read the labels on some of your food products you'll see these four letters: EGTA. EGTA [ethylenediaminetetracetic acid] is a commonly used chelator for keeping food fresh by chelating calcium and other ions to keep bacteria from dividing.) The problem is chelators can't cross the blood–brain barrier. Another problem is that chelators are not specific to a single molecule so they also take many that are essential for normal cell function. However, these problems are being solved through the development of new technological approaches (e.g., nanoparticle-conjugated metal chelators) that not only allow penetration of the blood-brain barrier but are more selective in the heavy metals to which they bind.

The Little Powerhouses that Shouldn't

There is strong evidence that oxidative stress plays an early role in the onset of Alzheimer's disease and so antioxidants have been an area of research focus since the 1990s (Figure 15.1). To understand this, a little background is required. If you ever took high school or college biology you'll likely know about the little powerhouses of the cell. This is the name given to mitochondria because they are the primary sites where ATP is generated. So these little powerhouse factories, or more correctly organelles, pump out ATP energy molecules that are needed for everything from cell division and movement to the transmission of nerve impulses. The problem is, as ATP is being generated, there are by-products that are generated. Like any factory making good stuff, there are always bad by-products and mitochondria are no different. The problem is the by-products are reactive oxygen species (ROS) that can really mess things up. So let's take a bit of a basic mitochondrial tour and in doing so enter the realm of reactive oxygen species and, as well, the hot topic of antioxidants.

Mitochondria are central to the survival of human cells. From an evolutionary point of view, they are a unique cell component because they originally were a bacterial type of cell that infected our cell line way back when life had barely emerged from the primordial ooze. So, as you might guess, mitochondria are quite complex. But to understand their role in Alzheimer's disease we only need to know or be reminded of a couple of basic points. As shown in Figure 15.2, each mitochondrion in the cell is surrounded by two membranes, cleverly called the inner and outer mitochondrial membranes. The inner membrane surrounds a matrix where the events of ATP formation begin, with some ATP molecules being made here. Other breakdown products drive what is called the electron transport chain (ETC) that resides in the inner mitochondrial membrane itself. This is where the good and the bad of ATP production occur.

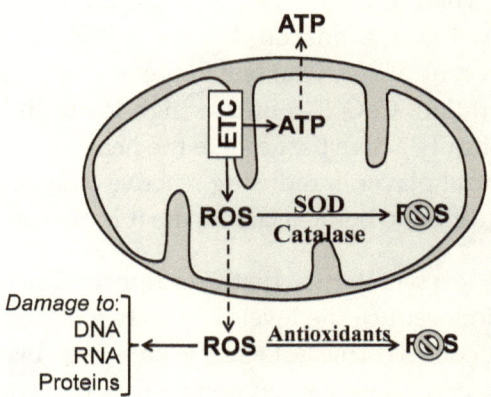

Figure 15.2. Antioxidants and mitochondria. ETC, electron transport chain; ROS, reactive oxygen species; SOD, superoxide dismutase.

As ATP is generated by the electron transport chain, reactive oxygen species are produced as shown in Figure 15.2. Reactive oxygen species are bad because they damage the cell's DNA, RNA and proteins as well as phospholipids and other molecules. Reactive oxygen species can leak out of the mitochondria and do so at higher levels in aging individuals and during certain diseases. Normally the cell gets rid of them by natural means. In the mitochondria and cytoplasm are natural antioxidant enzymes that remove reactive oxygen species. These enzymes are superoxide dismutase (SOD) and catalase. Usually these are sufficient to keep cells healthy by removing all excess reactive oxygen species. Our diet also helps keep reactive oxygen species at bay, especially diets rich in antioxidant vitamins such as E, C, carotenoids and the B vitamins (B6, B12 and folate). There is a relationship between aging and reactive oxygen species and so today antioxidant therapies are relatively widespread. However, our interest lies in the role of reactive oxygen species in Alzheimer's disease.

Pharmaceutical Antioxidant Therapies

There really aren't a lot of approaches that have been developed outside of using natural dietary routes to prevent or slow the progression of Alzheimer's disease. One of the central therapies is based on preventing reactive oxygen species formation in the first place, which of course is a logical way to begin. It involves one of the components of the electron transport chain called coenzyme Q_{10} or coQ_{10}. The coenzyme also goes by the name ubiquinone. For simplicity, like the ads on TV, we'll just call it CoQ. This coenzyme is a central and vital one in the electron transport chain for ATP generation. CoQ is found at high levels in the brain and other metabolically active tissues like the heart, liver and kidneys. It is also a central player in reducing reactive oxygen species levels because in addition to being a coenzyme it is also an antioxidant.

Several studies have shown that addition of CoQ can provide neuroprotection, reduce the levels of reactive oxygen species and stabilize mitochondria. This last effect is important because it means less reactive oxygen species can escape into the cytoplasm to do damage. Mitochondrial integrity is also important in preventing the death of brain cells. But there are problems with this approach, not the least of which is the fact that CoQ can't cross the blood–brain barrier (BBB). As an aside, this inability of drugs to cross the blood–brain barrier is a major problem that faces the development of any drug that has the brain as its target. The blood–brain barrier has evolved to keep things out of the brain except those things in the blood that are essential to its function. For CoQ, there's another equally complex problem. Normally, as its name implies, the enzymes in the electron transport chain are aligned in a precise sequence—a chain of enzymes that transport electrons. In the Alzheimer's brain the electron transport chain becomes disorganized. When it is disrupted, CoQ can't carry out its work as a coenzyme, leading to reduced ATP production.

Since CoQ has had some positive effects in treating Alzheimer's and other diseases, different chemical forms of it have been developed that will cross the blood–brain barrier. One of these, called MitoQ (aka triphenylphosphonium-linked CoQ), has been shown to cross the blood–brain barrier, inhibit reactive oxygen species formation, allow ATP to be formed, stabilize mitochondria and prevent nerve cell death. It also works in the disrupted electron transport chain of Alzheimer's brains and concentrates several hundredfold in cells thus increasing its potency. A lot of good attributes have set the stage for taking MitoQ from Phase II to Phase III trials in the future.

The biochemical pathway underlying CoQ synthesis is well studied, so that too may provide routes to developing new CoQ-related pharmaceuticals. As for other CoQ pharma approaches, only two antioxidants are on the horizon at present. ALCAR (actyl-L-carntine) and LA (R-α-lipoic acid) are under active study. So far combinations of these antioxidants have only been examined in dog, mice and rat models of Alzheimer's disease where they have been shown to reduce cellular insult by reactive oxygen species, maintain mitochondrial integrity and increase the number of mitochondria in the hippocampus.

Since oxidative stress due to mitochondrial dysfunction is considered as an early and possibly critical event in Alzheimer's disease. drugs are being developed to stabilize mitochondria. One of these, called "dimebon", binds a channel or pore in the mitochondria preventing leakage that leads to oxidative stress. However, the positive results from a successful small Phase II study with mild–moderate Alzheimer's subjects were contradicted by a subsequent large Phase III clinical trial. That said, controlling mitochondrial dysfunction continues to be focus for ongoing research.

Mitochondria are also central players in cell death. As such their role in the events of brain cell death that are linked to neurodegeneration, brain shrinkage and the increase in ventricular size ("holes" in the brain) is under intense scrutiny as well.

Some might wonder why the value of nutraceuticals and folk remedies were not discussed here or in previous sections. To date there is no compelling evidence that any nutraceuticals or folk remedy can slow the progression of Alzheimer's, let alone protect against it. Some of the Alzheimer's disease websites listed at the end of the references can provide the latest research on this and other topics related to this and other chapters in this book.

Anti-Inflammatory Drugs

Re-checking the above chart (Figure 15.1) will reveal that another therapy involves anti-inflammatory drugs. As their name implies, these drugs stop or prevent inflammation. As yet the role of inflammation in Alzheimer's disease is not well understood. That said, various anti-inflammatory pharmaceuticals have actually been shown to slow the progress of Alzheimer's disease not only in animals but also in people.

In Chapter 5 the cells of the brain were discussed, including microglia which are fundamentally the macrophages of the brain. These cells, along with reactive astrocytes, are involved in controlling inflammatory event in the brain. Several lines of evidence link activated microglia to the conversion of amyloid beta into its fibrillar form prior to plaque formation. They are also believed to cause excess glutamate release leading to excitotoxicity, a topic that is covered below.

There are two basic types of anti-inflammatory drugs: steroids and NSAIDs (non-steroidal anti-inflammatory drugs). Aspirin (acetylsalicylic acid) is the most commonly known NSAID but, sadly, it doesn't help with Alzheimer's disease to anyone's knowledge. However other NSAIDs, especially naproxen (also known as Aleve™ and by other names), initially had shown some success in Alzheimer's trials but subsequent research revealed they did not slow the progression of the disease. A similar story exists for Vioxx™ (rofecoxib). So, while some lines of research are still ongoing, no anti-inflammatory drug has proven to be effective at slowing the progression of Alzheimer's disease.

The Trend Away from Using Anti-Psychotics

People with Alzheimer's disease can suffer from a diversity of behavioral and psychological symptoms. These behaviors are often referred to as "acting out". They include aggression, agitation, and in the later stages of the disease, delusions and hallucinations. Typically the first response in such cases was to prescribe antipsychotic drugs or other medications to alleviate the symptoms. The trouble is antipsychotic drugs were developed to treat problems like schizophrenia, not Alzheimer's disease. More to the point, these drugs are not designed for long-term use in persons with dementia. Today there is a trend away from this drug therapy approach. Some countries, such as England and Wales, are developing strategies to decrease the use of pharmaceuticals in the treatment of the symptoms of Alzheimer's disease. In fact, England has made it a national priority to significantly reduce the use of antipsychotic drugs for people with dementia.

The goal now is to look for alternative ways to alter the negative behaviors associated with Alzheimer's disease. As discussed in Chapter 1, one way is to implement the factors that increase the quality of life and to decrease those factors that decrease the quality of life. In other words, providing a comfortable, stress-free environment for the person with Alzheimer's disease can reduce the triggers that elicit the negative behaviors associated with the disease.

Chapter 16

A Final View

To this point we've covered a lot of ground. For some, this may have seemed like an arduous journey with so many unknowns and such a diversity of less-than-friendly names and terms. The truth is we've only begun to break ground in the coal mine of darkness that is Alzheimer's disease. That said, many significant and helpful breakthroughs have been attained and more are on the horizon. Here we will summarize what we have covered in this book by presenting a more-or-less comprehensive model of how Alzheimer's is viewed today. Then we will look at why Alzheimer's occurs and some exciting new approaches that are the current focus of biomedical research.

A Basic Model for Alzheimer's Disease

A basic comprehensive model summarizing the key events and stages of Alzheimer's disease is shown in Figure 16.1.

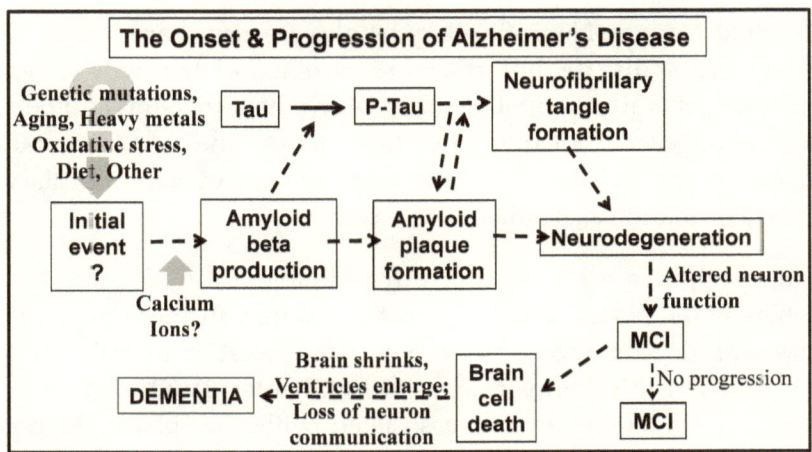

Figure 16.1. A model of the major events of Alzheimer's disease. MCI, mild cognitive impairment

Many questions remain about the cause, onset and progression of Alzheimer's disease. What is the initial event or events that lead to the disease? Clearly a primary factor is aging itself. But this alone is not sufficient. So research focus has been on the role of heavy metals, oxidative stress, diet and other causes which were touched upon in Chapter 15. It is important to note, however, that some of these (e.g., oxidative stress) may be a result of some other initial event rather than being the primary cause. As detailed in the following section on the much-reviewed "Calcium Hypothesis", calcium ions likely play a role in the early events of Alzheimer's. There is no doubt calcium ions are important in the disease but they may also be a later contributor that is involved more in nerve malfunction and degeneration. In the end, the key and earliest documented functionary is amyloid beta which, as detailed in Chapter 6, accumulates to form amyloid plaques.

Clearly, amyloid plaque formation is—to use a now overworked phrase—a "hallmark of Alzheimer's disease", as is the formation of neurofibrillary tangles. These events are believed to be the primary cause of the changes underlying the malfunction and ultimate death of neurons that result in the neurodegenerative events of the disease. The amyloid beta peptides, especially amyloid beta 42, coalesce with other components to form amyloid plaques. Neurofibrillary tangles are also characteristic of Alzheimer's disease but they are also associated with other neurodegenerative taupathies. It is widely held that amyloid beta formation and/or plaque formation initiate the events of tau hyperphosphorylation that starts the process of neurofibrillary tangle formation as detailed in Chapter 7.

Finally, there are intersecting ways (double arrow, Figure 16.1) whereby the plaque and tangle pathways may further interact in the neurodegeneration process. Neurodegeneration initially leads to mild cognitive impairment (MCI; Chapter 3). One's loss of memory and other events associated with this phase do not always progress. When they do, continued neurodegeneration can lead to neuronal death, an event linked to brain shrinkage, enlargement of brain ventricles ("holes"), and massive loss in neuronal communication. These events, and likely others, underlie the final decline into the dementia phase of Alzheimer's disease.

The Calcium Hypothesis

The major hypotheses for Alzheimer's disease were listed in Chapter 8 (Table 8.1). As mentioned in the previous section, one of these is the "Calcium Hypothesis". There is no doubt that calcium ions play a major role in Alzheimer's disease but it likely is a complex one since these ions function in so many essential life processes. An overwhelming body of scientific literature details the importance of calcium homeostasis and cell communication not only in neurons but in every cell in our bodies. Some of these are shown in Figure 16.2. For example, calcium is essential for cell division in all cells. It also regulates cell death (apoptosis). In nerves, it mediates neurosecretion, nerve impulse and membrane integrity. By binding to other proteins such as calmodulin, the primary calcium-binding protein of all cells, it also mediates a number of other functions such as learning and memory in normal brains. There is also evidence from a diversity of sources that calcium, interacting with calmodulin, mediates events of amyloid processing and turnover as well as tau phosphorylation (Chapters 7, 12).

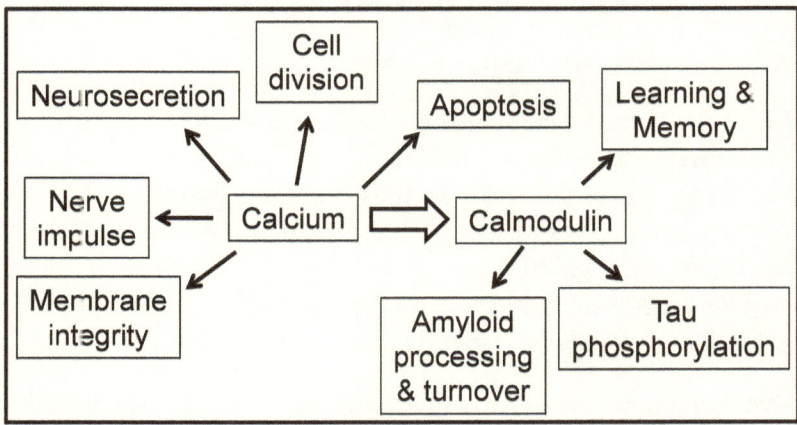

Figure 16.2. The "Calcium Hypothesis" of Alzheimer's disease is based on the loss of control on calcium levels in neurons. The unregulated levels of calcium negatively impact many processes that underlie the normal function and survival of neurons.

The levels of calcium inside neurons are tightly controlled in healthy cells through their movement across the cell membrane, by uptake and release from intracellular stores and from various calcium-binding proteins. Neuronal stimulation leads to increases in intracellular calcium levels that, in turn, lead to controlled secretion of neurotransmitters such as acetylcholine (Chapter 9) and glutamate (Chapter 10). The "Calcium Hypothesis" proposes that uncontrolled alterations to calcium levels, called calcium dysregulation, are an underlying cause of Alzheimer's disease. Like a leaky boat, nerve cell membranes in Alzheimer's brains allow calcium ions to flow in and overwhelm normal cell functions.

In support of this, there is evidence that increasing levels of intracellular calcium can drive the formation of some of the characteristic lesions such as the accumulation of amyloid beta. While increased calcium can affect amyloid beta peptide accumulation, the peptides in turn can further perturb calcium homeostasis, likely by forming unregulated pores in the cell membrane. Clearly the calcium hypothesis should and will be a central model for biomedical research but, while studies are ongoing, as yet no drugs are available on the market for controlling calcium function in Alzheimer's disease.

Early and Accurate Diagnosis Is Key

Most drug therapies are stage dependent and are primarily effective when carried out during the very early stages of Alzheimer's disease, so critical definition of these stages is essential. Defining the primary changes in the brain that signal the development of the disease is critical to diagnosing the onset of the disease. Much work on various biomarkers is underway as discussed throughout the book and detailed in Chapter 11.

Developing non-invasive but precise approaches for early detection will allow doctors to implement therapies that may significantly slow the progression of Alzheimer's disease. This will be of value to the person suffering from the disease plus their caregivers as well as society as a whole. Combining neuropsychological testing with other specific biomarkers such as cerebrospinal fluid analysis, brain imaging and genetics is the key. Many groups are working worldwide to establish and validate these criteria.

For example, if we include the staging used by some researchers to modify Figure 1.3 from Chapter 1, we can see that the additional stage of "severe cognitive disorders" (SCD) is inserted (Figure 16.3). This stage is believed by some to clarify earlier events of mild cognitive impairment (MCI) with more advanced changes (SCD) that are a prelude to full-blown dementia as detailed in Chapter 3. As researchers develop more precise staging, then it will be possible to glean more precise data from ongoing therapeutic research which will ultimately benefit everyone. In the meantime, there will be a state of flux as such staging is defined and agreed upon by all who do such research.

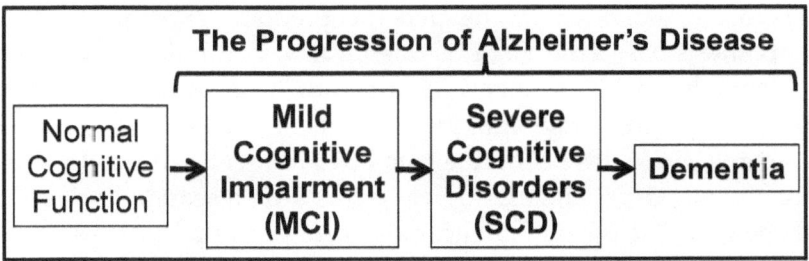

Figure 16.3. An example of stages in the progression of Alzheimer's disease.

While it's easy to criticize past research or to be frustrated with such issues as how to stage Alzheimer's disease, without such work we wouldn't know how to progress in the future. In short, doing research allows us to understand events, fine-tune approaches and clearly define what needs to be done next. It doesn't always lead to an immediate solution, but it is required if we ever hope to find one. Now, let's look in a bit more detail at the issues linked to simply understanding the early phases of Alzheimer's disease: mild cognitive impairment.

In 2012, a group of researchers analyzed the prevalence and incidence of mild cognitive impairment only to find that the definitions used to define this early stage of Alzheimer's disease varied significantly. They found that, in 42 different publications, there was no consistency in defining the early events of cognitive impairment—each study used a different way of categorizing exactly what mild cognitive impairment was. Without a consistent and precise definition of the stages or sub-types of mild cognitive impairment, it is fundamentally impossible to completely interpret the results of any therapeutic interventions. Thus it is possible that a drug may actually be quite effective if administered at one stage of mild cognitive impairment but not at another. In the absence of precise staging and by pooling all of the data, successful outcomes get diluted by unsuccessful or improperly interpreted results. This not only leads to erroneous conclusions about the efficacy of the therapy but it hides potentially beneficial results.

The Future of Alzheimer's Research

There are those that argue that the predominance of amyloid hypothesis-based research is taking away funding for other potentially viable avenues. Arguments have been made that because of the amyloidocentric view of Alzheimer's disease research, there has been little true advancement and no effective treatments. This suggests other avenues of research, especially those revealed by GWAS and multi-pronged approaches should be brought to the forefront of research. But as of the start of 2013, it is still not clear or agreed upon what those research areas should be.

It is not feasible scientifically or financially to study every line of evidence that comes up as a potential route to understanding the initiation and progression of Alzheimer's disease. What is needed is honest, data-driven guidance that allows Alzheimer's research to progress in a way that looks to the future rather than being mired in the past. That can only be determined by groups of both young and established scientists, working together on equal footing, whose sole goal is to find the causes and cures for Alzheimer's disease. So let's look at some novel approaches that are currently being taken.

How Low Can You Go?

There is a school of thought that it is fundamentally impossible to get to the basis of any disease without understanding the normal function of the proteins that are involved. Most disease proteins are also involved in normal life processes. This makes these proteins difficult to study because if you delete (knock out) the gene in animal models to see what it does, the result can be lethal. A paper was just published in the Journal of Biomedical Science that deals with this issue specifically in relation to the normal functions of huntingtin (Huntington's disease) and presenilin (Alzheimer's disease) in neurodegeneration. The interesting thing is this work promotes the use of cellular slime molds, little organisms that don't even produce nerve cells! While this may sound far-fetched to the layperson, it actually makes a lot of sense. Unlike humans and even mice, these little soil-based creatures are cheap, quick and easy to grow, mutate and genetically analyze, so dissecting gene and protein function is comparatively easy. Already that group had shown that huntingtin functions in fish by regulating the ability of cells of the future brain and spinal cord to stick together. So going lower on the evolutionary scale could provide unique insights into Alzheimer's proteins as well. This new knowledge could in turn lead to new routes to understanding the disease, its progression and even novel drug development.

Is Systems Biology the Answer?

As we have seen, Alzheimer's disease is complex. A typical disease is an abnormal condition of the human body that is characterized by a specific set of symptoms. In reality, no two people with Alzheimer's disease show exactly the same symptoms. Furthermore, when some symptoms appear similar in different people they still can vary widely in their severity, rate of onset and progression. This makes Alzheimer's more like a syndrome: a collection of signs and symptoms that defines the abnormal condition. This has led some frontline researchers to suggest that we should look at the disease as Alzheimer's syndrome. While this suggestion will undoubtedly be of major concern to biomedical researchers who study the disease, for those concerned about the disease it's just the old "toe-may-toe—toe-mah-toe" issue. Who cares what it's called or how a word is pronounced—it doesn't change anything. The tomato is still a tomato and Alzheimer's is still a killer disease.

On the other hand, for scientists studying Alzheimer's as a syndrome this will widen the focus of their research. Today for many diseases, including cancer, this approach falls under the heading of "systems biology". Systems biology is a rapidly emerging biology-based interdisciplinary approach to understanding basic problems in the life sciences as well as in biomedically related areas. It involves the mapping of interactions between genes, proteins and other molecules in the body that have been revealed by large-scale experimental approaches.

In Chapter 13, we looked at Genome-Wide Association Studies (GWAS). In systems biology this would just be one of the components that is involved in an analysis. Large-scale approaches to data collection have not only been linked to genome studies but many other areas as well. These include metabolomics (studies on metabolism), proteomics (protein profile changes), lipidomics (changes in lipid profiles) and neuroimaging/neurodynamics (e.g., PET scans) among many others. Massive amounts of data are accumulated through original studies or data mining of previously published works. The data are then analyzed by powerful computers through complex mathematical algorithms and other approaches to reveal specific interactions between these different aspects of human biology that are linked to Alzheimer's or other diseases.

The systems biology approach is possible in part due to the advanced computing power that exists today as well as due to the decades of pure research carried out by mathematicians who started out modeling comparatively simple events like enzyme reactions. Since a single gene mutation can have multiple downstream effects, this kind of research can yield novel insight into the links between those effects. This can guide researchers in developing specific therapeutic approaches as well as put them on the right path to identifying the initial changes that caused the disease in question.

Why Does Alzheimer's Exist?

While historically the focus has been on characterizing the classic lesions that define Alzheimer's disease—amyloid plaques and neurofibrillary tangles—there is still much to be learned. A big question is, "Why does Alzheimer's exist?" Answering this question could provide special insight in our fight against the disease. After all, the disease had to start sometime back in the history of humans if not before. Understanding how it first arose and how it became so insidious a disease would be useful information. In spite of this, there are only a few groups who are doing research on the evolution of Alzheimer's.

Is the disease just an inevitable result of aging? As we age, all body tissues and organs, as well as their functions, progressively decline. Shouldn't we expect the brain to do the same? The brain, like any other organ, is just a collection of cells. While the brain is a unique collection of cells, as we learned in Chapters 4 and 5, cells are just cells—each type specialized for the role(s) it performs in our bodies. One of the defining attributes of brain cells, especially neurons, is their unique ability to store information as memories and to help us learn from events we experience. Early in life, the brain is a flexible organ in the sense that its programming becomes modified through learning and life experiences. This kind of "neuroplasticity" is central to our lives, allowing us to adapt, express appropriate behaviors, recall events and socialize effectively.

There are those that believe this attribute of neuroplasticity, the ability of the brain to change and adapt, is costly because it wastes biochemical energy that is essential for the maintenance of our bodies. This, of course, is understood in terms of bioenergetic costs by those in the know. But the idea is that while the genes that drive brain function are beneficial in allowing the brain to function and change, by doing so they become a detriment through this high bioenergetic cost. The formal term is "antagonistic pleiotropy", which is one of many general evolutionary theories of aging.

As part of these concepts, the early accumulation of amyloid plaques and neurofibrillary tangles may actually have originated as a positive evolutionary solution. Some evolutionary biologists have suggested that the unhealthy accumulation of the soluble peptide amyloid beta, a peptide known to have many deleterious effects in cells, was coagulated into insoluble amyloid plaques to remove its harmful effects (Chapter 6). Early in our evolution, getting rid of amyloid beta in this way would have allowed brain cells to survive and function normally longer in life.

Now as lifetimes have increased, this positive feature has become a negative one. As more and more amyloid beta accumulates into plaques as we age and as they continue to grow, then these once positive storage sites now become toxic entities themselves. A comparative scenario exists for neurofibrillary tangles which might have served as ways to get rid of excess levels of phosphorylated tau (Chapter 7) inside of cells, allowing them to continue functioning normally. In the aging individual, the positive effect of sequestering phosphorylated tau becomes a negative as neurofibrillary tangles interfere with neuron function and survival. Thus, as human life expectancy increased, these originally beneficial evolutionary solutions turned into problems. Evolutionary approaches and interpretations are leading to insights in other ways as well.

Evolutionary Research, Medicine and Alzheimer's Disease

Along related lines, researchers are studying how specific genes (e.g., APOE) linked to the onset of Alzheimer's have evolved. These kinds of approaches have spawned an area of research called evolutionary medicine. The goal is to not only understand how genes have changed and affected cell function, but how the body's defense mechanisms (e.g., immune response) evolved in response to those changes. Underlying this is the quest to find the cause(s) of Alzheimer's disease. Researchers argue that because something like amyloid plaque accumulation is correlated with Alzheimer's disease doesn't prove that it is the cause. Thus, as mentioned above, plaques and tangles in fact may be defense mechanisms that initially serve a neuroprotective role.

One way to learn more about these issues is to do research on other species that form amyloid beta, amyloid plaques, phosphorylated tau and neurofibrillary tangles to reveal what effects they have in those organisms. This kind of research has shown, as expected, that aging monkeys and other primate species undergo changes in these constituents similarly to humans. Furthermore, those changes can lead to Alzheimer's-like symptoms similar to those seen in humans. What was less expected from this kind of research was that non-primate species, such as whales, dogs, rats, birds and fish, also produce amyloid beta and show age-related cognitive decline.

While it may seem unorthodox to many of us, these evolutionary approaches can offer fresh insight into the origin and progression of Alzheimer's disease. As a result, new therapies may be developed. These kinds of studies also reveal another important aspect of Alzheimer's disease: it's much more complex than we realize. The more we study it, the more we learn how much there is still to learn. The reality is, the only way to solve the riddle of Alzheimer's disease is to take any and all viable approaches that can give us the insight we need to find the causes and a cure.

The First Alzheimer's Patient Re-Examined

If anyone has any doubt that current biomedical research can find the causes and cures for Alzheimer's, it may be put to rest by the following. As we learned in Chapter 1, Dr. Alois Alzheimer described plaques and tangles and the neurological underpinnings of the disease that is named after him today. What we didn't learn is that the patient who helped shed light on this disease was Auguste Deter, who some consider to be one of the most famous patients in the history of medicine. While Alois and Auguste are long gone, it turns out that they have recently contributed new information on Alzheimer's disease.

Scientists uncovered the slides of Auguste's brain and verified the neurological changes that Dr. Alzheimer observed and recorded for posterity. But that was just the beginning. Auguste had early-onset Alzheimer's, originally known as pre-senile Alzheimer's disease. Genetics are known to play a role in this form of the disease, as was discussed in Chapter 12, so researchers extracted DNA from those prepared slides to determine if any risk genes had the appropriate mutations. While APOE variant epsilon 4 was normal, the gene for presenilin-1 (PSEN1) had the Alzheimer's disease form of the mutation. Thus Auguste Deter's Alzheimer's was likely a result of her having the presenilin-1 mutation. As if this weren't enough, these results also suggest that researchers could go back through old medical records and isolate DNA from a diversity of brain sections from a diversity of patients to gain further insight into the genetics behind Alzheimer's disease.

The Future Holds Hope

There is no doubt the Alzheimer's population is growing daily. The search for causes and a cure seems like a daunting task. While the historical biomarkers of the disease, the presence of amyloid plaques and neurofibrillary tangles, still dominate the research and pharmaceutical landscape there are many who believe these are but reflections of more pertinent underlying causes. Just what are those causes? Nobody knows. As we have seen, there are many candidate "at risk" genes and proteins but none of them stand alone as the "cause" of Alzheimer's disease. In fact, recent research would argue that whatever causes the disease plays its role decades before any symptoms or markers of the disease become manifest. The other outcome of research is that none of the current drugs that are designed to slow the progression of the disease are globally effective. While some improvement is seen in some individuals with some of the drugs, there is no statistical evidence that any drug is effective at the population level. This does not mean that that there is no hope.

While it might seem that there is a negative undertone to ongoing work based on the inability to offer any short-term hope, in the longer term both the cause and cure will result from research. This is because legions of dedicated biomedical researchers worldwide are looking in every nook and cranny to find them. Many years ago, getting a malignant cancer was basically a death sentence but today a vast deal is known about the diversity of cancer types and specific therapies have been developed to treat them. So while an all-encompassing cancer cure has not yet been discovered, the underlying causes are quite well understood and effective therapies exist for many types of the disease.

So we might think of our understanding of Alzheimer's disease to be equivalent to our understanding of cancer a decade or so ago. While this might not seem too encouraging, the existing approach to understanding diseases is advancing at a phenomenal rate. Not only that, researchers are thinking about Alzheimer's disease more as a syndrome, a range of diseases, rather than a single disease with a single cause. Applying all the current arsenal of research weapons from genomics, proteomics and metabolomics along with newly conceived systems biological and evolutionary approaches is rapidly providing unique insight into Alzheimer's disease. More importantly, improved methodologies are being applied in pharmacological studies and therapies are being undertaken which will shortly lead to greater therapeutic assistance for Alzheimer's sufferers and their caregivers.

Selected References

Note: These are general categories to assist the reader in finding additional resources. Since most of the references are review articles many different aspects of Alzheimer's disease are also covered in most of them.

Biomarkers

Cummings, J. L., 2011. Biomarkers in Alzheimer's disease drug development. Alzheimer's & Dementia 7: e13–e44.

Hampel, H., S. Lista and Z.S. Khachaturian, 2012. Development of biomarkers to chart all Alzheimer's disease stages: The royal road to cutting the therapeutic Gordian Knot. Alzheimer's & Dementia 8: 312-336.

General Articles on Alzheimer's Disease

Alzheimer's Association Report, 2012. Alzheimer's disease facts and figures. Alzheimer's & Dementia 8: 131-168.

Castellani, R., et al., 2010. Alzheimer disease. Disease Monthly 56: 484-546.

Hebert, L.E., et al, 2013. Alzheimer disease in the United States (2010-2050) estimated using the 2010 census. Neurology (online prior to printing: http://www.neurology.org/content/early/2013/02/06/WNL.0b013e31828726f5)

Sperling, et al, 2011. Toward defining the preclinical stages of Alzheimer's disease: Recommendations from the National Institute on Aging-Alzheimer's Association workgroups on diagnostic guidelines for Alzheimer's disease. Alzheimer's & Dementia 7: 280-292.

Terry, Jr., et al, 2011. Alzheimer's disease and age-related memory decline (preclinical). Pharmacology, Biochemistry and Behavior 99: 109-210.

Warda, A., et al, 2012. Mild cognitive impairment: Disparity of incidence and prevalence estimates. Alzheimer's & Dementia 8: 14-21.

Wortman, M., and W. Wimo, 2011. Alzheimer's disease international: Making dementia a global health priority. Alzheimer's Disease International Conference, Toronto, Canada. (available at: http://www.alz.co.uk/adi-conference-2011-presentations)

WHO Report, 2012. Dementia: A public health priority. WHO and Alzheimer's Disease International, UK.

Genetics of Alzheimer's Disease

Bettens, K., K. Sleegers and C.V. Broeckhoven, 2013. Genetic insights into Alzheimer's disease. Lancet Neurology 12: 92-104.

Borovecki, F., et al, 2011. Unraveling the biological mechanisms in Alzheimer's disease—Lessons from genomics. Progress in Neuro-Psychopharmacology & Biological Psychiatry 35: 340–347.

Contestabile, A., F. Benfenati, and L. Gasparini, 2010. Communication breaks-Down: From neurodevelopment defects to cognitive disabilities in Down syndrome. Progress in Neurobiology 91: 1–22.

Fleisher, A.S., et al, 2012. Florbetapir PET analysis of amyloid-β deposition in the presenilin 1 E280A autosomal dominant Alzheimer's disease kindred: a cross-sectional study. Lancet Neurology 11: 1057-1065.

Goate, A. and J. Hardy, 2012. Twenty years of Alzheimer's disease-causing mutations. Journal of Neurochemistry 120: 3-8.

Guerreiro, R.J., D.R. Gustafsonc and J. Hardy, 2012. The genetic architecture of Alzheimer's disease: beyond APP, PSENs and APOE. Neurobiology of Aging 33: 437-456.

Jonsson, T. et al, 2012. A mutation in *APP* protects against Alzheimer's disease and age-related cognitive decline. Nature 488: 96-99.

Knickmeyer, R.C., et al, 2013. Common variants in psychiatric risk genes predict brain structure at birth. Cerebral Cortex (ePub: PMID: 23283688).

Ruiz, A., et al, 2013. Exploratory analysis of seven Alzheimer's disease genes: disease progression. Neurobiology of Aging 34: 1310e1-1310e7.

Schellenberg, G.D. and T.J. Montine, 2012. The genetics and neuropathology of Alzheimer's disease. Acta Neuropathol. 124: 305-323

The ENCODE Project Consortium, 2012. An integrated encyclopedia of DNA elements in the human genome. Nature 489: 57-74.

Neuroimaging

Li, Q-T and L-O. Whalund, 2011. The search for neuroimaging biomarkers of Alzheimer's disease with advanced MRI techniques. Acta Radiologica 52: 211-222.

Peterson, R.C., 2011. Alzheimer's disease neuroimaging initiative (ADNI). Alzheimer's Disease International, Toronto, 2011.

Reiman, E.M. and W.J. Jagust, 2012. Brain imaging in the study of Alzheimer's disease. NeuroImage 61: 505-516.

Sakoglu, U., et al, 2011. Paradigm shift in translational neuroimaging of CNS disorders. Biochemical Pharmacology 81: 1374-1397.

Smith, K., 2012. fMRI 2.0. Nature 484: 24-26.

Pharmaceutical and Other Therapeutic Approaches

Chavez, S.E. and D. H. O'Day, 2011. Calmodulin binds to and regulates the activity of beta-secretase (BACE1). Chapter 10, pp 128-136 In: Marissa R. Boyd, ed. "Alzheimer's Disease Diagnosis and Treatments". Nova Biomedical, NY.

Corbett, A. and C. Ballard, 2012. New and emerging treatments of Alzheimer's disease. Expert Opinion on Emerging Drugs 17: 147-156.

Danysz, W. and C.G. Parsons, 2012. Alzheimer's disease, β-amyloid, glutamate, NMDA receptors and memantine—searching for the connections. British Journal of Pharmacology 167: 324-352.

Fazil, M., et al, 2012. Nanotherapeutics for Alzheimer's disease (AD): Past, present and future. Journal of Drug Targeting 20: 97-113.

Galimberti, D. and E. Scarpini, 2011. Disease-modifying treatments for Alzheimer's disease. Therapeutic Advancements in Neurological Disorders 4: 203-216.

Ihl, R., et al., 2011. World Federation of Societies of Biological Psychiatry (WFSBP) guidelines for the biological treatment of Alzheimer's disease and other dementias. The World Journal of Biological Psychiatry 12: 2-32.

Lukiw, W.J., 2012. Amyloid beta (Aβ) peptide modulators and other current treatment strategies for Alzheimer's disease (AD). Expert Opinion on Emerging Drugs 17: 43-60.

Liu, W., F. Dou, J. Feng and Z.Yan. 2011. RACK1 is involved in β-amyloid impairment of muscarinic regulation of GABAergic transmission. Neurobiology of Aging 32: 1818–1826.

Luo, X. and R. Yan, 2010. Inhibition of BACE1 for therapeutic use in Alzheimer's disease. International Journal of Clinical and Experimental Pathology 3: 6-18-628.

Malinow, R., 2012. New developments on the role of NMDA receptors in Alzheimer's disease. Current Opinion in Neurobiology 22: 559-563.

Mullane, K. and M. Williams, 2013. Alzheimer's therapeutics: Continued clinical failures question the validity of the amyloid hypothesis—but what lies beyond? Biochemical Pharmacologys 85: 289-305.

Müller, U., P. Winter and M.B. Graeber, 2013. A presenilin 1 mutation in the first case of Alzheimer's disease. Lancet Neurology 12: 129-130.

Nathanson, N., 2008. Synthesis, trafficking and localization of muscarinic acetylcholine receptors. Pharmacology & Therapeutics. 119: 33-43.

Probst, G. and Y.-z. Xu, 2012. Small molecule BACE inhibibitors: a patent literature review (2006-2011). Expert Opinion in Therapeutic Patents 22: 511-540.

Salomone, S., et al, 2012. New pharmacological strategies for treatment of Alzheimer's disease: focus on disease modifying drugs. British Journal of Clinical Pharmacology 73: 504-517.

Small, G. and R. Bullock, 2011. Defining optimal treatment with cholinesterase inhibitors in Alzheimer's disease. Alzheimer's & Dementia 7: 177–184.

Stone, J. G., et al, 2011. Frontiers in Alzheimer's disease therapeutics. Therapeutic Advances in Chronic Disease. 2: 9-23.

Sun, X., K. Bromley-Brits, and W. Song, 2012. Regulation of β-site APP-cleaving enzyme 1 gene expression and its role in Alzheimer's Disease. Journal of Neurochemistry 120: 62-70.

Tayeb, H.O., et al, 2012. Pharmacotherapies for Alzheimer's disease: Beyond cholinesterase inhibitors. Pharmacology and Therapeutics 134: 8-25.

Vellas, B., et al, 2011. AMPA workshop on challenges faced by investigators conducting Alzheimer's disease clinical trials. Alzheimer's & Dementia 7: e109-e117.

Yiannopoulou, K.G. and S. G. Papageorgiou, 2013. Current and future treatments for Alzheimer's disease. Therapeutic Advances in Neurological Disorders 6: 19-33.

Plaques and Tangles

Carter, C.J., 2011. Alzheimer's disease plaques and tangles: Cemeteries of a pyrrhic victory of the immune defence network against herpes simplex infection at the expense of complement and inflammation–mediated neuronal destruction. Neurochemistry International 58: 301-320.

Chavez, Sara E. and D. H. O'Day, 2007. Calmodulin binds to and regulates the activity of Beta-Secretase (BACE1). Alzheimer's Disease Research Journal 1: 37-47.

Glenner G. G. and Wong C. W. (1984a) Alzheimer's disease: initial report of the purification and characterization of a novel cerebrovascular amyloid protein. Biochemical and Biophysical Research Communications 120: 885–890.

Glenner G. G. and Wong C. W. (1984b) Alzheimer's disease and Down's syndrome: sharing of a unique cerebrovascular amyloid fibril protein. Biochemical and Biophysical Research Communications 122: 1131–1135.

Hirokawa, N. 1991. Molecular architecture and dynamics of the neuronal cytoskeleton. In pp 5-74. The Neuronal Cytoskeleton, RD Burgoyne (ed.), Wiley-Liss, New York.

Liu, L., et al, 2011. Trans-Synaptic Spread of Tau Pathology *In Vivo*. PLoS One 7: e31302

Lopes, J.P. and P. Agostinho, 2011. Cdk5: Multitasking between physiological and pathological conditions. Progress in Neurobiology 94: 49-63.

Ludovic, M., X. Latypova, and F. Terro, 2011. Post-translational modifications of tau protein: Implications for Alzheimer's disease. Neurochemistry International 58: 458–471.

Martin, L., et al, 2013. Tau protein kinases: Involvement in Alzheimer's disease. Ageing Research Reviews 12: 289-309.

Morris, M. et al. 2011. The Many Faces of Tau. Neuron 70, 410-426.

O'Day, D. H. and M. A. Myre, 2008. Alzheimer's Disease: The Calmodulin Connection and β-Amyloid. pp. 1-10. In "Alzheimer's Disease Research Trends", pp. 1-10, Ed. A.P. Chan, Nova Biomedical, NY.

Zhang, H., et al, 2012. Proteolytic processing of Alzheimer's β-amyloid precursor protein. Journal of Neurochemistry 120: 9-21.

Quality of Life

Banerjee, S., B. Gurland and N. Graham, 2010a. Improving quality of life for people with dementia: The ADI-Stroud symposia. Alzheimer's Society of the UK conference, 2011. (available at: http://www.alz.co.uk/adi-conference-2011-presentations)

Banerjee, S. et al, 2010b. The Stroud/ADI dementia quality framework: a cross-national population-level framework for assessing the quality of life impacts of services and policies for people with dementia and their family carers. International Journal of Geriatric Psychiatry 25: 249-257.

Mossello, E. and E. Ballini, 2012. Management of patients with Alzheimer's disease: pharmacological treatment and quality of life. Therapeutic Advances in Chronic Disease 3: 183-193.

Various and New Research Approaches

Di Domenicoa, F., et al, 2012. Quantitative proteomics analysis of phosphorylated proteins in the hippocampus of Alzheimer's disease subjects. Journal of Proteomics 74: 1091-1103.

Glass, D.J. and S.E. Arnold, 2012. Some evolutionary perspectives on Alzheimer's disease pathogenesis and pathology. Alzheimer & Dementia 8: 343-351.

Camardola, S. and M.P. Mattson, 2011. Aberrant subcellular neuronal calcium regulation in aging and Alzheimer's disease. Biochimica et Biophysical Acta 1813: 965-973.

Juhasz, G. et al, 2012. Systems biology of Alzheimer's disease: How diverse molecular changes result in memory impairment in AD. Neurochemistry International 58: 739-750.

Li, Y.F., et al, 2011. Phosphodiesterase-4D knock-out and RNA interference-mediated knock-down enhance memory and increase hippocampal neurogenesis via increased cAMP signaling. Journal of Neuroscience 31:172-183.

Mancuso, C.,et al, 2102. Natural substances and Alzheimer's disease: From preclinical studies to evidence based medicine. Biochimica et Biophysica Acta 1822: 616–624.

Mastroeni, D., et al, 2011. Epigenetic mechanisms in Alzheimer's disease. Neurobiology of Aging 32: 1161–1180.

Mizwicki, M.T., et al, 2012. Genomic and Nongenomic Signaling Induced by $1\alpha,25(OH)2$-Vitamin D3 Promotes the Recovery of Amyloid-β Phagocytosis by Alzheimer's Disease Macrophages. *Journal of Alzheimer's Disease* 29: 51-62.

O'Day, D. H. and M. A. Myre, 2004. Calmodulin Binding Domains in Alzheimer's Disease Proteins: Extending the Calcium Hypothesis. Biochemical Biophysical Research Communications 320: 1051-1054.

Myre, M., 2012. Clues to γ-secretase, huntingtin and Hirano body normal function using the model organism *Dictyostelium discoideum*. Journal of Biomedical Science 19: 41.

Schneider, L.S., 2012. Ginkgo and AD: key negatives and lessons from GuidAge. Lancet Neurology 11: 836-837.

Vellas, B., et al, 2012. Long-term use of standardized ginkgo biloba extract for the prevention of Alzheimer's disease (GuidAge): a randomized placebo-controlled trial. Lancet Neurology 11: 851-859.

The Alzheimer's Epidemic Website

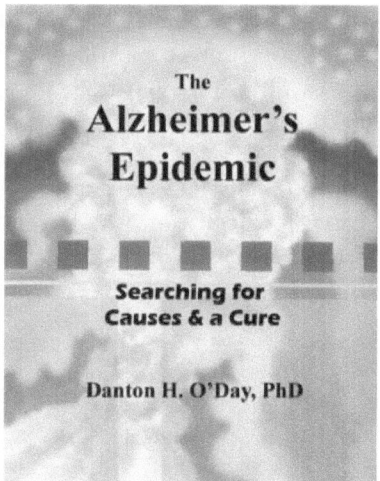

www.AlzheimersEpidemic.com

❖ Download free PowerPoint slides of figures from the book
❖ Download free animations of many figures from the book plus others
❖ Plus free book updates and the latest information on Alzheimer's disease

Some Official Alzheimer's Disease Websites
(not in any specific order)

www.alz.co.uk/ A global voice on Alzheimer's

www.alzheimers.org.uk/ Alzheimer society in the UK

www.alz.org/ Alzheimer association in the USA

www.alzheimer-europe.org/ Alzheimer society in Europe

www.alzforum.org/ A forum based on latest Alzheimer's disease research.

www.adni-info.org/ A research sharing site on neuroimaging

http://www.alzhh.ca/ Alzheimer society of Brant, Haldimand Norfolk, Hamilton and Halton)

http://www.alzheimer.ca/en Alzheimer's Society of Canada

FYI: Appropriate Alzheimer's Websites

Appropriate Alzheimer's disease websites will usually be designated as .org, .edu, or .net. Others may be indicated by their country of origin (e.g., Alzheimer.ca). Many governments and universities offer information about the disease as well so one can go to these website and search. Websites that are designated as .com, .biz are more likely to be designed to sell products related to Alzheimer's disease and are more likely to offer product-specific information rather than unbiased content. It is important to check out more than one source of information especially when "cures" or "new effective treatments" are suggested.

About the Author

Danton H. O'Day, PhD, is professor emeritus in both the Department of Biology at the University of Toronto Mississauga and the Department of Cell & Systems Biology, at the downtown campus of the U of Toronto. He has published well over 120 original, refereed research articles and edited many books. He has co-authored several articles and book chapters on novel aspects of amyloid beta processing in Alzheimer's disease. With over 40 years teaching experience in Canada and the US, he wrote this book as a guide for non-scientists on the research being done to understand, control and someday cure Alzheimer's disease.

eBooks by the Author:

The Human Cell — The Unit of Life & Disease
(ISBN-13: 978-1-4566-0970-2)

Human Developmental Biology
(ISBN-13: 978-1-4566-1008-1)

Co-authored with Aldona Budniak:

How to Succeed at University — International Edition
(ISBN-13: 978-1-4566-0941-2)

How to Succeed at University — Canadian Edition
(ISBN-13: 978-1-4566-0876-7)